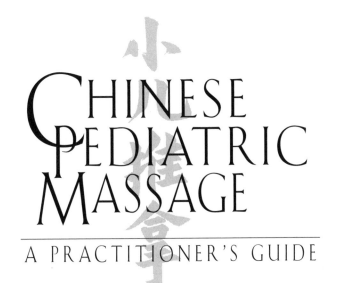

CHINESE PEDIATRIC MASSAGE

A PRACTITIONER'S GUIDE

CHINESE PEDIATRIC MASSAGE

A PRACTITIONER'S GUIDE

Techniques and Protocols

for Treating Childood Illnesses

and Chronic Health Problems

KYLE CLINE, LMT

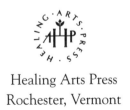

Healing Arts Press

Rochester, Vermont

Healing Arts Press
One Park Street
Rochester, Vermont 05767
www.InnerTraditions.com

Healing Arts Press is a division of Inner Traditions International

Note to the reader: *This book is intended as an informational guide. The remedies, approaches, and techniques described herein are meant to supplement, and not to be a substitute for, professional medical care or treatment. They should not be used to treat a serious ailment without prior consultation with a qualified health care professional.*

LIBRARY OF CONGRESS CATALOGING-IN-PUBLICATION DATA

Cline, Kyle, 1957–
Chinese pediatric massage ; a practitioner's guide / Kyle Cline.
p.   cm.
Includes bibliographical references and index.
ISBN 0-89281-842-5 (alk. paper)
1. Massage for children—China.   2. Massage for infants—China.   3. Medicine, Chinese.   I. Title.
RJ53.M35 C58 2000
615.8'22'0830951—dc21   99-049254
CIP

Printed and bound in the United States

10   9   8   7   6   5   4   3   2   1

Text design and layout by Virginia L. Scott
This book was typeset in Goudy with Usherwood and Schiedler initials as the display typefaces

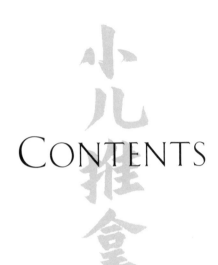

CONTENTS

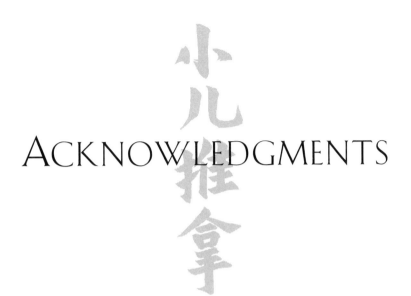

ACKNOWLEDGMENTS

ANY BOOK OF THIS SCOPE IS THE FINAL PRODUCT of many people's efforts. While I take responsibility for any errors, credit is due to many more people than would fit on this page.

In China I wish to acknowledge the many generations of doctors whose efforts have culminated in the current practice of Chinese pediatric massage. I would also like to acknowledge the generous help and support of my teachers and friends: Dr. Huang Da-gang, Dr. Li Hong-wai, Dr. Zheng Shou-jie, Dr. Shen Yang-he, Dr. Lin Li, Dr. Ye, Dr. Ting Ji-feng, Wu Jun-miao, Nurse Lu, Ye Jing, and Antoine Eid.

In the United States I acknowledge the invaluable help of my teachers and colleagues: Bob Flaws, Honora Wolfe, Master Mantak Chia, Maneewan Chia, Subhuti Dharmananda, Dr. Edythe Vickers, Dr. Zhang Qing-cai, Judith Rose, Peggy Nauman, and Wing K. Leong.

I greatly appreciate the support and assistance provided by the staff of Healing Arts Press, especially Peri Champine, Susan Davidson, Jeff Euber, Jon Graham, Virginia Scott, and copy editor Laura Matteau.

Finally, my deepest appreciation to the many children and parents, both Chinese and American, who have contributed to my understanding of Chinese pediatric massage.

Feedback or Questions

I appreciate any feedback or questions you may have. You can write to me at P.O. Box 10714, Portland, OR 97296. You can also reach me by e-mail (kyle@healartspro.com).

For videos and other learning materials about Chinese pediatric massage, please see appendix G: Recommended Resources.

Kyle Cline, LMT

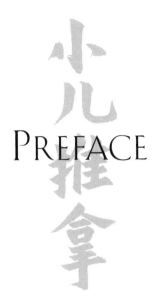

PREFACE

SINCE THE EARLY 1970s ACCEPTANCE OF traditional Chinese medicine (TCM) in the United States has grown in several distinct phases. When China reopened its doors to the West, acupuncture was the first aspect of TCM to gain popular attention. Later, as U.S. practitioners expanded their overall knowledge of TCM, Chinese herbal therapy also came to be practiced here. The third branch of TCM has received less attention in the West. This branch, tui na, is the use of massage or hand manipulations for an energetic effect on the body. Beyond these three main branches, there is also growing interest in tai qi, qi gong, and dietary therapy.

Why the slow recognition of tui na? First, it takes years of strong dedication to training and practice to become a skilled tui na practitioner. Also, massage in the West is defined differently than in China. There a practitioner of tui na is considered a doctor on the same level as an acupuncturist or an herbalist. In the United States, this same practitioner is considered less qualified to treat people and is confined to a limited scope of practice.

Chinese pediatric massage (CPM) is an even lesser-known specialty within tui na. However, as more Western practitioners expand their knowledge and practice, tui na and pediatric massage should become more common. My hope in this book is to provide a thorough and complete Chinese pediatric massage reference. The amount of information and the scope of practice will, I believe, support pediatric massage as a distinct professional modality.

Pediatric massage may be much easier for Western practitioners to adapt than adult tui na. The basic pediatric techniques are relatively easy to learn and apply, and the points and theory represent only small variations from the common foundation of TCM concepts.

In the United States children face many health challenges due to lifestyle, environmental conditions, and the overwhelming use of pharmaceuticals in the health care system. When children do become ill, the usual reliance on antibiotics and other potent drugs may achieve dramatic short-term results at the expense of overall health and balance. CPM is, for many conditions, a viable alternative as either a primary treatment or a complement to other therapies. Learning pediatric massage will allow practitioners more flexibility in choosing the course of treatment that is the least invasive and has the fewest side effects. By embracing the concepts of Chinese medicine and the treatments of pediatric massage, a different approach to the overall health care of children may be offered.

Pediatric massage can be used by Western practitioners to expand the overall care of patients and their families. In doing so you may bring a fuller appreciation of a complete, holistic vision of health to people who can benefit from it.

Notes on Translation
氣

When TCM material is introduced from China, it is important to recognize two issues regarding translation. First is the language translation from Chinese to English. Second is the translation of a therapeutic modality from a Chinese to a Western cultural and social context.

Language Translation

The many differences between the Oriental and Western cultures are easily appreciated through their respective languages. These differences in worldview and reality are firmly rooted in the structure and usage of language. Although technical translation from Chinese to English may be relatively easy, attempting to convey the essence of the material is another matter. In the case of this book, the subtleties required me to make several decisions.

This book is not a direct translation of any one Chinese work on pediatric massage. Rather, it is a synthesis of the literature available at this time, direct teachings from Chinese and Western practitioners, and my own clinical experience. Because I am writing for practitioners, I assume you have familiarity with the general concepts of Chinese medicine.

In general the Chinese put much less emphasis than westerners on book learning, preferring to learn the subtleties of tui na through practical experience with a teacher. This is reflected in the lack of availability and fragmented nature of most pediatric massage literature. One book provides useful protocols with little information on assessment. Another provides useful assessment information, but only a few points and protocols. Several books include massage as but one therapy out of many used in pediatrics. I am attempting to bring all of the related pediatric massage information into one reference.

In doing so I have tried to incorporate as much information and detail as possible. Unusual or seldom-used techniques, points, and protocols are included to present as comprehensive a reference as possible. While some information, such as the torticollis (wryneck) protocol, may not currently seem relevant here, no one knows what the future may bring.

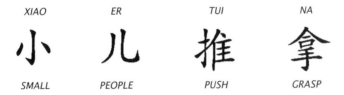

Xiao er tui na is translated here as "Chinese pediatric massage." A technical translation of this phrase might be "pediatric energetic hand manipulations" or, better yet, "pediatric tui na." Still, I have chosen the term *Chinese pediatric massage* to convey the intent of this treatment while recognizing the need to make it understood in a Western society. With due appreciation and respect for the tui na profession, these words in themselves will probably never have the meaning in the United States that they have in China. In China, technically, tui na is not considered massage, for it is in a professional field distinct from the common, ordinary concept of folk massage. However, in the U.S. there is simply no equivalent term to convey this concept of energetic, medically oriented physical manipulations.

In general I have limited the use of pin yin transliteration for several reasons. First, unless a practitioner is fluent in Chinese, the use of pin yin creates a barrier to understanding the meaning of a concept or word. There are some exceptions—qi, yin, yang, and so forth—which are difficult to translate and are included in appendix E: Glossary of Chinese Medical Terminology. Second, pin yin is a somewhat arbitrary choice for transliterating Chinese characters into Arabic letters. The profusion of written materials on Chinese arts has created much confusion, because different transliteration methods have been used. (For example, *chi* also appears as *qi* and *ch'i*.) Again, this confusion gets in the way of true understanding of the material. It is difficult enough to truly grasp Chinese medical concepts without such additional obstacles.

Capturing the essence of the pediatric materials in English requires a certain amount of poetic license to interpret the intent. While this may lead to subjective judgments, it is inevitable when disciplines are brought across cultural borders. It can be compared to the process of a skilled practitioner learning foundation material and then making it his or her own through practice. This process involves defining and making subjective judgments according to the practitioner's personality and the context in which he or she practices. This does not detract from the professional field; it is a sign of growth and development.

The translation of pediatric massage technique names is much the same. In the English sources consulted, a single technique might be described by totally different names (for example: pinching, fingerneedling, nipping). Also, a similar name (such as kneading) might be used to describe totally different hand movements. To a Western reader unfamiliar with the subtle terrain of Chinese English, the confusion would be yet another obstacle to learning the material. The English names I have chosen for techniques are thus intended to describe the nature of the hand movement as simply and descriptively as possible.

Another technical translation issue concerns points. Pediatric points have never been Westernized by substituting a number for the Chinese name. In this book I use English translations of the Chinese names to encourage you to become familiar with the *character* of the point, which is generally reflected in its name. There is some controversy, however, over which point-name translations are technically correct. For this book I selected the point names that most clearly reveal the character of the point. *Grasping the Wind* (Ellis 1989), for instance, is used for pediatric points that coincide with acupuncture points. I have taken other point-name translations from a variety of sources.

My final note on translation involves capitalization. Only point names are capitalized. TCM terminology, conditions, and patterns are not capitalized in the text, because these words have become a normal part of practitioners' daily language.

Language translation is full of controversy and potential for misunderstandings. Rather than shy away from this process for fear of making mistakes, this book is published with the hope that it is of practical use to practitioners. The refinement of concepts, words, and names is an ongoing process that reflects the growing nature of our profession. This book is not the final word on Chinese pediatric massage, but I hope it is a useful step toward a growing body of TCM knowledge in the United States.

Therapy Translation

Although the language translation from Chinese to English is difficult, much more difficult is the task of translating the practice of Chinese medicine onto Western soil.

Common sense dictates that the practice of pediatric massage in the United States cannot literally be the same as in China. Too many factors differ for the same therapy to be applied exactly the same way in both cultures, including social, economic, political, medical, environmental, dietary, and lifestyle conditions.

Given a few decades of perspective, it is clear that acupuncture has been subtly adapted to meet the needs and conditions found in the United States. Currently it seems that the practice of Chinese herbology is also undergoing a similar process. The same will hold true for Chinese pediatric massage. Certainly the foundations and basic understandings of pediatric massage will remain constant. But how practitioners choose to apply this modality to children in the U.S. will be determined by the context of their practices and who they are. Only an awareness of this cultural translation process will allow us to remain true to the original intent and body of pediatric massage knowledge, while at the same time respecting Western cultural standards and issues. This process will not weaken Chinese pediatric massage, but instead will enliven it.

How to Use This Book

As with acupuncture and herbal reference books you need not read this book page by page, attempting to memorize all the information. There are too many details and your retention rate would likely be marginal. A more reasonable approach would include the following steps.

Read chapters 1 through 5, History through Assessment. This will provide background information and an overview of CPM. Much of this information should be familiar to Oriental medicine practitioners, with some variations due to children's energetic immaturity.

Read appendix A: Technique Practice on a Rice Bag. Make a simple rice bag to practice hand techniques.

Read chapter 6, Techniques, for an overview, particularly the section on the four requirements for good technique. Also see appendix B, Chinese Pediatric Massage Core Information, for a list of basic techniques. You will want to practice these on the rice bag. This requires time. Daily practice of ten to fifteen minutes is more valuable than one hour of practice once a week. With patience and time the techniques will become easier, smoother, and more relaxed. Solicit feedback from an instructor or a practitioner familiar with the tui na style of hand techniques. Videos of techniques are also available; see appendix G; Recommended Resources.

Appendix B, Chinese Pediatric Massage Core Information, includes a list of basic

points. Choose five to six points to study at a time. Borrow a child friend to practice locating these points. Remember—use the rice bag to gain proficiency before practicing on children!

Appendix B also has a list of basic protocols. Study one protocol at a time. Practice the sequence of each protocol repeatedly on the rice bag and include variations on technique and points.

With several months of regular practice, the core material outlined in appendix B should be fairly easy for you. As you begin to see children in practice you can research other points, techniques, and protocols as needed.

The appendixes contain additional information that may be helpful: traditional Chinese medicine terminology, Chinese herbs for pediatrics, pediatric points grouped by categories, and point names cross-referenced by English name, pin yin name, and acupuncture number.

The indexes are arranged to help you locate techniques, points, protocols, and internal herbal formulas as easily as possible.

Pediatric massage requires time and patience. A practitioner must have basic theoretical information, clear assessment skills, working knowledge of points, skill in performing hand techniques, and understanding of how it all fits together in a treatment. Most of all, proficiency in pediatric massage requires practice and experience. I hope that this book will aid you in the process.

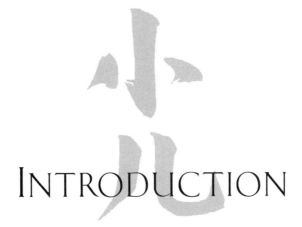

INTRODUCTION

CHINESE PEDIATRIC MASSAGE IS A USEFUL THERAPY for children from birth to approximately twelve years old. There is some controversy regarding the upper age limit. However, most authorities agree that CPM is most effective from birth to age six. After that you must assess the child carefully to determine his or her relative energetic maturity. Practitioners frequently combine aspects of pediatric and adult tui na.

Pediatric massage is a valuable addition to the repertoire of any practitioner because it is a simple extension of common Chinese medicine concepts applied to children. At the same time it is a distinct specialty within Chinese medicine because children present a different energetic framework than adults. These differences are apparent in all aspects, from energetic anatomy and physiology through assessment, points, and treatment. Thus, in this book I will assume that you already have a firm understanding of TCM theory and practice, and will focus on those adaptations necessary given the differences presented by children. The theories of pediatric massage offer clear guidelines on these differences for assessment and treatment.

Massage techniques offer health care practitioners a unique and valuable alternative. On many occasions treatment options for children are limited, or prove so invasive or strong that they create unnecessary side effects. Pediatric massage techniques offer a way to influence the energetic qualities of the child without the invasiveness of other modalities. This usually proves to be much more tolerable to the child, easier on the parent, and more effective in the long term.

The role of pediatric massage in China today is varied, depending on the location and available health care resources. Most of the established TCM hospitals and schools have a department of tui na that includes a pediatrician. While there is a long history of pediatric massage in China, its development has been sporadic and uneven across the entire country. It is apparent, however, that pediatric massage is an integral part of the overall medical system in China.

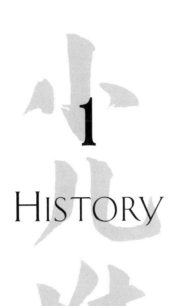

1

HISTORY

ALL WRITTEN WORK ON CHINESE MEDICINE makes reference to the historical literature that conveys the subject's background and development. Pediatric massage is no exception.

The historical record of Chinese medicine spans three to five thousand years—a distinct obstacle in its sheer vastness. Surviving written materials are few; the passage of time and societal changes resulted in the loss of important works. Much of the TCM historian's work must be a process of deduction, of piecing limited information into a coherent picture. Many of the original books have been lost; however, these classics are often referred to in surviving texts. Unschuld (1985) in *Medicine in China* gives exemplary insight into the social, economic, and political forces that shaped the development of Chinese medicine. It is a valuable book for understanding the ground from which TCM grew.

No single date can be conclusively identified as the beginning of pediatric massage. Like most aspects of Chinese medicine CPM evolved slowly but steadily into its present form. Like the other medical branches it has gone through a series of phases ranging from flourishing advancement to outright repression and near extinction. During this rocky development it has endured everything from official government recognition and support to a secretive underground status among committed practitioners. It is important to understand the general trends of this development to fully appreciate where pediatric massage has arrived today.

Although there are some references to pediatric massage dating back to the *Nei Jing* (The Inner Classic), the earliest available written literature is from the Sui/Tang dynasty (A.D. 581–907). Sun Si-miao in *Prescriptions Worth a Thousand Gold* discussed a dozen infantile diseases, including convulsions, nasal blockages, night crying, and abdominal distension. For each condition he outlined gao mao therapy, which combines external herbal preparations with hand techniques.

During the Song dynasty (960–1279) Qian Zhong-yang differentiated pediatric syndromes, energetics, diagnosis, and treatment. This work was published in three volumes as *Key to the Treatment of Children's Diseases*. During the same dynasty Liu Fang wrote *A New Book for Child Care*.

Reflecting CPM's development in the Yuan dynasty (1279–1368), a pediatric massage department was established in the Institute of the Imperial Physicians. At this time the tui na department was divided into two major branches: bone setting and pediatrics.

The Ming dynasty (1368–1644) was a period in which CPM advanced and indeed flourished. At this time it was organized into an academic discipline within medical institutions. Pediatrics was recognized as a specialty practice within the massage field. Major clinical and theoretical advances occurred during this dynasty, including an independent system of pediatric diagnosis, hand techniques, points, and protocols.

Many books have survived from the Ming period. In 1575 Zhou Yu-fan's clinical manual, *Secrets of Infantile Tui Na Therapy*, included a fifteen-step protocol for physical examination of children. In 1601 Yang Ji-zhou authored *Compendium of Acupuncture and Moxibustion*, with a section by Chen—Infantile Remedial Massage—devoted to pediatrics. Chen's work included descriptions of hand techniques and treatment regions; he emphasized diagnosis, especially through the index finger venule. In 1604 Gong Yun-lin expanded on Chen's work in the illustrated *Guide to Infantile Tui Na Therapy*. In 1676 Xiong Yun-ying wrote a three-volume work titled *General Descriptions of Infantile Tui Na Therapy*. Also at this time, Luo Ru-long wrote a five-volume treatise on *The Essentials of Tui Na Therapy*. Other books written during this time period include *The Canon of Massage for Children*; *The Complete Classic of the Secret Principles of Massage to Bring Infants Back to Life*; *Secret Pithy Formula of Massage for Children*; *Classics of Tui Na for Children*; *Secrets of Tui Na and Pulse Taking for Children*; and *Secrets of Tui Na for Infants*.

During the Qing dynasty (1644–1911) several classic works were written before political change made the environment increasingly oppressive to Chinese medicine. In the early and middle parts of the Qing dynasty Cheng Fu-zheng wrote *A Complete Book of Pediatrics*; Xiong Ying-siong wrote *Elucidations of Massage for Children*; Xia Yun-ji wrote *The Massage for the Care of Infants*; and Zhang Zhen-jun wrote *Revised Synopsis of Massage*. In 1888 Chang Chen-chun revised Zhou's Ming dynasty book as *A Course of Infantile Tui Na Therapy*.

The later Qing dynasty saw major breakdowns throughout the social, political, and economic structures of China. These also had a significant impact on the practice of medicine. During this time Chinese medicine, not enjoying government support, was taught as a family tradition—the father teaching the son. From the mid-1800s on many medical practices became dispersed and disorganized.

This situation changed significantly when, after the Communist Revolution (1949), the government decided to reorganize and promote traditional Chinese medicine. Many scattered and separate pieces of classical Chinese medicine began to be re-formed into a coherent whole. Pediatric massage was considered a valuable aspect and was included in this reorganization. Thus, during the 1950s it enjoyed a resurgence in popularity and organizational development.

Chinese history, however, is full of contrasting and opposing shifts. The advancements made in the 1950s were followed by the declines of the Cultural Revolution in the late 1960s and early 1970s. As during the Qing Dynasty, but for a much shorter time period, TCM experienced little development. The writing and publishing of medical works was halted, and many books were destroyed. Teachers and practitioners were barred from their work and forced to pursue other types of labor. It is difficult to know how much was lost during this period, for the Chinese are only now beginning to acknowledge what happened during the Cultural Revolution.

In 1979 the policies of the Cultural Revolution were lightened and slowly, TCM began rebuilding. Pediatric massage continues to this day to be a significant aspect of the complete system presented by traditional Chinese medicine.

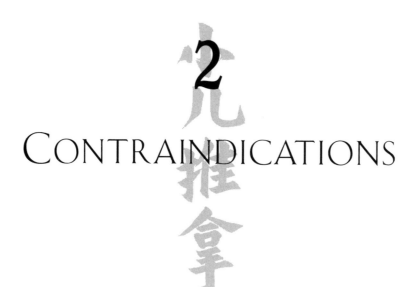

2
CONTRAINDICATIONS

MOST OF THIS BOOK IS DEVOTED TO explaining when and how to use massage with children. However, the first decision a practitioner must make is whether it should be used at all.

The guiding principle behind any decision to treat or not is *First, do no further harm.* This is a very commonsense approach to evaluating the child's condition and the effect of the proposed treatment. A corollary is to consider contraindicated any condition that you do not clearly understand or feel qualified to deal with. Referral to an appropriate practitioner or specialist may be the most valuable "treatment" available.

No list of contraindications can cover every possible clinical situation; however, if we are guided by the above principles, the task of evaluating each child becomes easier.

Following are some common contraindications for massage in general and pediatric massage in particular (this list is not exhaustive):

- Unknown diagnosis
- Directly on tumors, acute skin diseases, open wounds, or skin trauma (burns)
- Notifiable acute infectious diseases (hepatitis, tuberculosis, diphtheria, typhoid fever)
- Internal hemorrhaging
- Children taking heavy medication (particularly analgesics)
- Spinal cord trauma

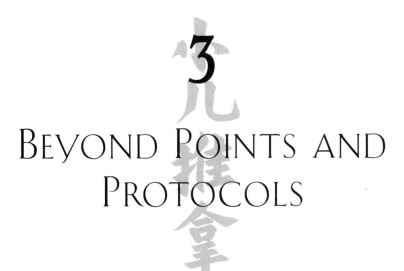

3
BEYOND POINTS AND PROTOCOLS

Treatment Environment
氣

The environment for massage should be warm, clean, and conducive to performing the treatments. It is useful to have pillows for the child to lie on, blankets to stay warm, and possibly a chair for a parent to sit and hold the child. An appropriate working surface, such as a massage table, is necessary. The height of the table is an important factor in the performance of hand techniques. A table with adjustable height is ideal.

Clothing
氣

In general it is advisable to keep the child clothed except for the immediate treatment area. This is especially important after you work on the abdomen.

Hygiene
氣

The practitioner should observe good hygiene. This requires hand washing before and after treatments and regular maintenance of trimmed fingernails in order to not interfere with performing techniques.

Massage Medium

An appropriate massage medium should be available and easily accessible. (See appendix F for massage mediums.) In the course of a treatment you should frequently replenish the medium on your fingers and hands. Place the medium in a spillproof container with a large opening that has easy hand access.

Touch

It is crucial that you employ an appropriate level of touch. The strength of your technique should be firm, but not painful for the child. This is a subtle skill that must be developed with regular and consistent practice on a rice bag. (See appendix A for rice bag practice details.)

Positioning

In order to perform techniques on various parts of the body, you must position the child in a manner both comfortable for him or her and conducive to your performance of the technique. In the course of a treatment the child may need to be repositioned frequently, possibly with assistance from a parent. Positioning the child must be done in a firm but gentle way. Sometimes it is advisable to have a parent hold the child in the lap for reassurance while a technique is performed. This should only be done when it does not interfere with technique, however.

Demeanor

Your demeanor as you relate with the child is very important. When possible it is beneficial to earn children's trust by talking and relating with them in a respectful manner. Children respond positively to adults who pay attention and relate to them as people. If children are old enough to communicate, explain what is happening and why. Be responsive to their reactions to the massage, asking for and respecting feedback. While techniques are performed, it may be useful to sing songs, share jokes, or tell stories in order to gain their confidence.

Posttreatment Attention

After you complete the massage, follow up on any questions the parent or child may have. This is a good time to reinforce preventive, dietary, lifestyle, or other suggestions that will improve the condition. Make sure that the child is well clothed and protected from wind, cold, and damp before he or she leaves. If it is feasible, discuss with the parent some basic massage techniques and points to perform at home.

Prevention

One of the most valuable contributions that Chinese medicine offers Western culture is its emphasis on working with disharmonies at a relatively subtle level, before they manifest as symptoms or disease. Whenever possible, discuss with children and parents what they can do to prevent recurrence of the condition, not just respond to its presence. Good preventive care will vary with each condition and individual. Think clearly about the condition and its roots, and give simple and realistic suggestions.

Diet
氣

Diet is a crucial component of the overall Chinese medical perspective on pediatric care. Bob Flaws, in several of his books (see appendix G, Recommended Resources), presents a very clear and compelling case for the importance of diet in pediatric preventive and therapeutic care. A complete discussion of diet is beyond the scope of this book. I recommend the above references and others to incorporate this aspect into pediatric care.

In general, because of the inherently deficient nature of spleen and stomach functions, suitable types and natures of food can play a critical role in the overall health of the child. Avoiding the extremes of hot, cold, and greasy foods, as well as practicing moderation in all food choices (especially sugars and dairy products), is important. With some awareness, parents who can monitor their child's food intake will notice correlations between certain eating habits and the onset of chronic problems (runny noses, earaches, and the like). Advising parents from a Chinese dietary viewpoint could play an important role in the overall treatment plan.

Lifestyle

The term *lifestyle* encompasses everything in children's lives that affects their energetic functions. In assessing adults you would inquire about work stress, relationships, emotional balance, and sexual health. With children you should also inquire about lifestyle, differing from adults only in the details. It is important to shift assessment perspective from an adult view and learn to see the world from the child's eyes. Lifestyle issues affect children as obviously as adults, and it is important to include these elements in your overall assessment and treatment.

Parents

Communicating well with the parents or caretakers is critical to the overall success of a treatment. Take as much time as necessary to gain the trust and compliance of the parents; children can sense the lack of these and become less cooperative. Each parent needs something different from the practitioner. Some may want to know how assessments are made and points selected; others might wonder about your amount of professional training. In any case, parents are entrusting their child to you, and it is important that a trusting relationship evolve. Educating parents is often as important as treating children. Many parents will respond positively to assisting in some way, either during the treatment or at home. Encourage them to be involved, and notice how this affects the children.

Treat the Mother to Treat the Child
氣

The Chinese medicine adage Treat the mother to treat the child emphasizes the strong connection between mother and child. In a literal sense, especially with breast-fed newborns, the nourishment of the mother is directly passed on to the child. However, in an energetic sense this relationship continues without or beyond the breast-feeding years. In addition to this dynamic is the congenital energetic foundation passed from parents to child. Clearly many of the parents', and particularly the mother's, energetic patterns will play a significant role in the child's life. Sometimes the most direct and effective way to treat the child is by treating the mother.

Practitioner Training

Your effectiveness as a practitioner will of course depend largely on your skills in pediatric massage. However, the study and practice of massage are primarily technique oriented. You must also pay significant attention to cultivating your own internal qi development. It is one thing to intellectually understand the concepts of qi, assessment, and so on; it is another to experience these in a clinical situation and be able to influence other people's energetic patterns. An ongoing qi gong practice is thus an important aspect of your continuing education.

4
ENERGETIC PHYSIOLOGY AND PATHOLOGY

THE DEVELOPMENT OF CHILDREN'S ENERGETIC SYSTEMS is similar to that of their structural and physiological systems. At birth each of these systems is immature, although functional at the level necessary for continued growth. The younger the child, the more immature the energetic system and the greater the difference from an adult's. For these reasons you must realize that a child is not simply a smaller version of an adult. Nor do all children present a single energetic physiology. The term *child* covers a wide spectrum of energetic differences. Unless specifically identified, the word *child* in this book is used in this general way.

The details of applying massage to a specific child must be adapted to fit his or her age—that is, you must account for the child's level of energetic physiology and of energetic pathology, then incorporate these into your assessment and treatment. I have thus divided this chapter into pediatric energetic physiology and pathology. General TCM principles apply, although in this book only those areas unique to children are presented.

Energetic Physiology
氣

An infant begins life with a soft body build; insufficient qi and blood; unformed tendons, blood vessels, and meridians; unstable shen; weak defensive qi; and immature essential organ qi.

Yin/yang theory describes the child as having insufficient yang while yin is not fully produced. *Yin* refers to body materials (essence, blood, fluids); *yang*, to internal organ functions. Due to immature yin and yang, neither the material base nor the energetic function of children is fully developed or capable.

Vitality and Growth

With appropriate congenital foundation and postnatal care, infants grow readily. Their physical build and energetic functions develop vigorously. In the first year children develop more rapidly than in later stages. In that first year, for example, they may grow more than two times in height and three times in weight; they also develop the capacity to turn over, sit, crawl, stand, and walk. This vigorous growth indicates the predominance of yang qi, which characterizes children's general energetic tendency.

Classical Chinese pediatric theory describes the normal course of growth and development as a process of "changing and steaming." *Changing and steaming* describes conditions of imbalance between yin and yang that manifest in fever, irregular pulses, and perspiration. These episodes generally resolve in a few days without treatment and are considered normal. *Changing* refers to the transformation of the five yin organs and occurs once every thirty-two days (ten times in one year). *Steaming* refers to the transformation of the six bowels induced by accumulated heat and occurs once every 64 days (nine times in 576 days). These are considered ordinary events and should not be seen as an illness. However, if children have not been properly cared for during these changing and steaming periods, they may become more susceptible to illness.

In addition to the changing and steaming process, children commonly experience conditions such as crying, fever, appetite loss, vomiting, and diarrhea. Periodic episodes of these conditions are considered normal. If the condition is a natural result of the child's body adapting and changing with the environment, it will usually resolve in a few days without treatment. If the symptoms last longer or become a regular, patterned response to certain environmental conditions, treatment may be indicated.

Common illness (such as vomiting, diarrhea, and fever) and normal childhood diseases (such as measles and chicken pox) will generally present very quickly and dramatically. Usually these conditions are easily changeable and may seem worse than adult conditions. This is because the child's reserves of qi, blood, and fluids are limited; strongly taxing diseases quickly exhaust all reserves.

The mutable nature of children is easily observed through their pulse, behavior, and response to illness. Several factors contribute to this dynamic, including inherent organ deficiencies and excesses.

Organ Deficiencies

At birth the meridians and internal organs are incompletely formed or, if complete, not totally strengthened. The spleen, lung, and kidney are especially delicate. As the child grows, the normal development process includes strengthening these delicate organs. Given proper postnatal care these organs will produce no endogenous pathological conditions in themselves. However, improper care can easily affect them.

SPLEEN

Normal spleen functions produce ample qi and blood, rich muscles, and vigorous growth. Children consume large amounts of ying qi for their constant growth and development, placing a heavy demand on spleen function. Because of this, improper feeding will easily cause illness.

The spleen is responsible for the transportation and conversion of food into qi. Prior to birth the infant relied on the mother's spleen function to provide food essence. Birth signals the beginning of this organ's functioning—and stress.

LUNG

The lung depends on the vigorous function of the stomach and spleen for strength and resistance to disease. Since the stomach and spleen function weakly in children, the lung also is weak.

The lung controls the qi of the entire body. Prior to birth this organ had developed but was not functional. Birth is also the beginning of the responsive functioning and stress of this organ.

KIDNEY

Children's growth and development, resistance to disease, and specifically bone, marrow, hair, ears, and teeth are all closely associated with kidney function. The kidney is indeed in charge of bones and marrow and serves as the congenital foundation of health, growth, and development. At birth the kidney takes on a large role in the responsibilities of body growth and development from the mother. Because of these large demands, kidney qi is often insufficient.

Inherent Excesses

In conjunction with the above organ deficiencies, children manifest several inherent excesses: heart qi, yang qi, and liver yang qi.

HEART

The excess fire of the heart may by a contributing factor to the overall unstable nature of the child's shen. *Shen* is defined as the spirit that provides guidance and foundation for the physical and energetic aspects of the child. Given the inherent hyperactive nature of the heart, and the deficient qualities of its partner organs, it is easy to see how shen becomes unstable. Unstable shen is obvious in the child's emotional manifestations, which so quickly shift from one extreme to another, like the wind on a blustery day. This is a normal aspect of childhood and should not be considered pathological (although possibly difficult to deal with). Other normal examples of unstable shen include a short attention span and self-centeredness.

Another factor to consider regarding unstable shen is how easily it can be startled. Extreme fright is particularly unsettling to shen that is already unstable. Classical Chinese pediatrics strongly emphasizes fright as a pathological factor to minimize and also to account for in the course of assessment and treatment. Shen strongly upset by fear may not see the smooth and easy transition to balance that is characteristic of less extreme emotions. The resulting pathological condition manifests in a variety of ways, but fright and unstable shen are the precipitating factors.

YANG QI

Energetically, the status of yang qi gives a general description of the active physiological aspects. In children the excessive quality of yang qi is reflective of their need for the basic physiological functions of transformation and change. From birth each child is involved in a constant process of transforming and changing energetic and physical structures. This is the general role of yang qi. In addition, in order for yin structure to develop, the yang transforming function of qi must be very strong.

The physical and energetic development of a child is very demanding. The general motivating force behind this transformation is, again, excessive yang qi.

LIVER YANG QI

A more specific example of the growth and transformative process involves liver yang qi. Like yang qi, liver yang qi is inherently excessive in children. Whereas excess yang qi presents a general motivating force, excess liver yang qi presents more specific functions.

The liver's function of blood storage and regulation has a major impact on the availability of nourishment to the body. The child's body is in a constant growth process with a very strong need for nourishment from blood.

Similarly, the liver function assists the stomach/spleen digestive process, playing a significant role in the assimilation of nourishment through food.

The liver's control of sinews relates to the body's capacity for movement. Much of the child's physical development is geared toward coordination of movement and body activity. A strong liver function is necessary if a child's physical activity and motor development are to reach a high level.

In a more general sense the liver's overall function corresponds to the wood phase (of the five phases). This phase is reflective of growth, much like tree sap rising. The liver provides a child with the resoluteness and drive to move forward, powering the incredible pace and rate necessary for growth and development.

Energetic Pathology
氣

In general children's pathological conditions are due to delicate internal organs, weak defensive qi, insufficient qi and blood, and weak meridians, skin, and muscles. The younger the child, the more susceptible to illness. This is because of the relative immaturity of the organs and their functions.

These factors lead to organ-deficiency patterns, excess patterns, changing syndromes, and seasonal disorders. Because children present a predominantly yang energetic foundation, these general patterns can quickly change and are sometimes unpredictable.

Due to the immaturity of yin and yang, the transformation of patterns occurs easily. For example, early-stage diarrhea often presents as an excess-heat syndrome due to retention of damp heat in the stomach and intestine. Continual heat retention easily consumes immature yin fluids, thus injuring yin. Conversely, deficient spleen qi or restrained spleen yang caused by damp can lead to yang injury. Due to the interdependence of yin and yang, injury to both yin and yang may occur.

Organ-Deficiency Patterns

The inherent energetic deficiencies of the spleen, lung, and kidney produce the following general pathologies.

SPLEEN/STOMACH

The child's large demand for qi produced by the spleen/stomach function can easily lead to digestive-related disorders. Due to its immature state, the spleen is required to produce food essence under conditions that are very demanding. Given proper care and support, development will proceed at a fast pace. However, improper diet or feeding as well as exposure to external pathogens can easily upset this delicate balance, manifesting in digestive and eliminative symptoms.

Spleen deficiency can easily lead to injury in the presence of improper feeding, hot or cold diets, or external pathogenic invasions (EPIs). As a result clear yang fails to rise, turbid yin fails to descend, and stomach qi is disharmonious. These conditions reflect in gastrointestinal distress, abdominal pain or distension, belching, vomiting, diarrhea, and malnutrition.

LUNG

Insufficient lung qi and weak defensive qi can lead to easy invasion by external pathogens and impair the lung functions in dispersing and descending. Patterns involving the common cold, coughing, asthma, and pneumonia may occur.

Because the lung is responsible for the skin and hair, its inherent deficiency in children results in weakness at the juncture between the skin and muscles. This important defense to EPIs is not compact enough to resist external invasions. This condition is especially noticeable if seasonal influences predominate and attack the lung at this level. The result may be impediments to the lung functions of ventilating and descending. Patterns of accumulated heat, fullness in the chest, productive cough, and dyspnea may result.

KIDNEY

The inherently deficient nature of the kidney, aggravated by improper postnatal care (and possibly congenital deficiencies), can lead to failure to nourish bones, marrow, and tendons. Thus, development will be impeded. Concurrent deficiency of kidney/liver yin may result in atrophy, developmental retardation, or flaccidity. In conjunction with deficient kidney/liver yin, excessive liver yang may produce wind. Liver wind can rise in the presence of heat or fire, resulting in convulsions, twitch, or opisthotonos.

Excess Patterns

The inherent excesses of heart, yang, and liver qi produce the following general pathologies.

HEART

The inherent excess of heart qi is most notable in the unstable nature of shen. Pathologies related to this dynamic may include emotional, spiritual, or physical imbalances. Unstable shen may also be a contributing factor to patterns originating from an extreme emotion, and these can influence the energetic function of any organ. For example, extreme fright might impact the unstable shen to such an extent that the heart is affected, resulting in night crying. The influence of extreme emotional situations could extend to almost any pattern of disharmony.

YANG QI

The inherent excess of yang qi is general and does not reflect in any specific pathologies, yet it does have a strong influence on the nature and course of most disharmonies. The quick, dramatic presentation and the adaptability of pathologies are related to excess yang qi. A rapid transformation of syndromes from one aspect to its opposite can be ascribed to how easily excessive yang qi is exhausted, and the resulting lack of corresponding yin balance.

LIVER QI

Excessive liver qi is similar to excessive yang qi pathologies in that it can create rapid changes in the child's energetic balance. Quick and strong emotional behaviors, such as shouting and anger, reflect a liver qi condition. However, emotions in general are ruled by the liver. The free flowing of any emotional qi is a sign of balanced liver qi. Conversely, the repression, stagnation, or denial of emotions can produce difficult behavior and physical conditions.

Liver yang rising may manifest as headaches, uncontrollable temper or anger, disturbed sleep, or irritability. Internal liver wind may produce nervous tics or convulsions. Liver qi invading the stomach or spleen may produce irritability, abdominal conditions, constipation and/or diarrhea, tiredness, gas, or vomiting.

Changing Syndromes
氣

The nature of children's diseases is likely to change rapidly from cold to heat and excess to deficiency. This is because of the basic unstable relationships among the organs and their functions due to their immature development.

Excess/Deficiency

In general a deficiency condition signifies insufficient healthy vital qi, while an excess condition signifies predominance of pathogens. The change from excess to deficiency may occur quickly or evolve into a complicated combination of the two.

Heat/Cold

During external pathogen attacks children generally manifest an excess-heat syndrome. As their vital qi becomes depleted this changes into a deficiency/cold syndrome. Once established the disease may transform quickly from an initial excess to a deficiency condition.

Seasonal Disorders

Due to the child's immature yang and defensive qi, external pathogens can easily penetrate the exterior. Seasonal climatic changes can thus have a large impact on children until they mature sufficiently to strengthen their defensive qi.

Quick Recovery and Response to Treatment

The combination of inherent deficiencies and hyperactive excess is the predominant feature of pediatric pathology. Overall, children are full of vitality; when imbalanced, their reactions are sensitive and prompt. The predominance of yang in children is responsible for the rapid development and changes in an illness. It is also responsible for children's vigorous growth, development, and strong ability to recover quickly.

Relative to adults, children's diseases are often simpler, showing less variety in signs as well as fewer emotional swings and multiple disease patterns. Because of their vigorous physiological functions, children can quickly marshal strong internal energetic resources. Given appropriate care they often exhibit a rapid recovery and response to treatment.

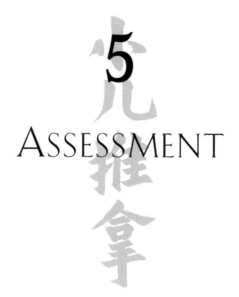

5
ASSESSMENT

ASSESSMENT IS A CRUCIAL COMPONENT of a pediatric massage treatment. An accurate assessment is the first step toward developing treatment principles and then a treatment plan.

The process of pediatric assessment has some points in common with adult assessment. The same major areas are covered. However, they have been adapted to accommodate the energetic differences of the child. You should also consider any Western medical tests or determinations in your overall assessment.

Pediatric assessment is accomplished by the four examinations: observing, listening, inquiring, and palpating. Of these, observation and palpation are probably relied on more than the others. This is because children are relatively unable to communicate subtle signs and symptoms. Listening symptoms may not always present during the examination. The inquiring phase should be actively pursued with both the child and the parent or caretaker, and as much information gleaned from them as possible. Remember that information from parents is secondhand; do not rely on it as heavily as you would self-reports from adults on their own conditions.

Observing
氣

Observation plays a key role in pediatric assessment. The child's exterior reflects any organ disorders clearly because the skin and muscle are tender and respond to stimulation easily. The quickly changing nature of the child requires that observation assessments be carried out quickly and throughout the entire treatment; you should continually notice changes and correlations. Such observation provides you valuable information on the child's prognosis and the strength of his or her constitution.

Your observations should include at least ten areas: tongue, index finger venule, complexion, face areas, Mountain Base, eyes, nose, ears, lips and mouth, and fingernails.

Shen

One of the most important and obvious aspects to observe is the shen, or spirit, of the child. Usually, a child's shen is not remarkable unless it is extremely strong or weak. A normal level of shen indicates a strong constitution and a relatively good prognosis, even if the condition is serious. What is immediately more noticeable is a child whose shen is dull. Observing the child as a whole (including behavior and actions) will give a clear picture of shen. The eyes are a particularly good indicator. Strong shen is reflected in clear, bright eyes and an outward manifestation of vitality. A dull shen is reflective of a more serious condition of weakened qi and will require a deeper level of treatment.

Index Finger Venule (IFV)

Observation of the index finger venule (IFV) is a supplementary assessment to pulse palpation in children younger than four to five years old. It dates from the Tang dynasty (A.D. 618–907).

The palmar index finger is divided into three segments named Wind Pass (proximal segment), Energy Pass (middle segment), and Vital Pass (distal segment). To observe the condition of the IFV, hold the child's finger such that the length of the palmar aspect is exposed. With one or two fingers, push gently from distal to proximal along the three segments to make the vein evident. The venule usually appears at the knuckle joints, not at the fleshy areas. It can be observed either on the palmar or lateral aspect of the index finger. Using cold water or alcohol can bring the IFV into more clarity.

IFV ASSESSMENT

This assessment method is primarily used to ascertain the severity, depth, and nature of an external pathogen, and whether digestive difficulties are hot or cold.

The length of the vein is reflective of the overall severity of the condition and how deep into the body disruption occurs. The color of the vein indicates the hot/cold and excess/deficiency nature of the condition.

The IFV assessment can be valuable, especially when you are attempting to assess very young children. However, you should not rely on it alone for a complete assessment; you must correlate it with other signs and symptoms.

Complexion

The five basic colors of the complexion—blue, red, yellow, white, and dark—each correspond to an internal organ or are reflective of internal conditions. Complexion colors are useful for distinguishing between excess/deficiency and hot/cold. Some of the observable colors of the complexion can be quite subtle. Observing in natural light and taking your time with the examination can produce a more accurate assessment.

Facial Areas

One facial area of particular importance is Mountain Base (Shan gen). This is the area roughly corresponding to Yin Tang (X 2) in adult acupuncture. The location is superior to the bridge of the nose and between the eyebrows. Mountain Base is a good indicator of the condition of the stomach/spleen. A bluish vein or tint at Mountain Base is indicative of a deficiency of stomach/spleen or liver wind.

Five Sense Organs

The tongue is the outward manifestation of the heart and can also show general signs of excess/deficiency and hot/cold.

The ears are the outward manifestations of the kidney and reflect the condition of the gallbladder meridian, which passes through this area.

The lips and mouth are the outward manifestations of the spleen and can reflect its condition.

The eyes, as the outward manifestation of the liver, are a clear indicator of that organ's condition.

The nose is the outward manifestation of the spleen and gives a clear reflection of that organ.

TONGUE

Sign	Pattern
Light red, free motion, moist	Normal
Delicate, tender, and moves easily	Normal
Thin white coating	Normal
Pale	Qi and blood deficiency
Thin white coating	EPI or cold
Moist	Cold damp
Thick white coating	Damp phlegm
Thin gray coating	Light EPI
White sticky coating	Internal cold damp
Bright red	Interior heat
Dry yellow coating	Excess internal heat or depleted fluids
Red, hard, and cracked	Upward invasion of toxic heat
Thick black coating	Strong EPI
Yellow; child plays with tongue, is chronically ill	Pathogenic invasion of stomach
White border, dry coating, and black center	Critical condition
Deep red or crimson	Ying qi and blood invaded by pathogenic heat
Purple	Qi and blood stagnation
Yellow sticky coating	Damp heat or turbid damp in middle burner
Yellow, dirty, and sticky coating	Food or milk retention
Dry peeled coating	Deficient kidney yin or fluid exhaustion
Pale red with disseminated red spots	Flaring heart fire
Dim purple	Qi/blood stagnation and stasis
Fat	Accumulated damp phlegm, fluid retention, or accumulated heat in upper body
Retracted	Blood deficiency or interior heat
Swollen, rigid	Convulsions
Child plays with tongue	Heart fire
Wagging	Heart wind fire
Scorched yellow	Heat stagnation
Greasy yellow	Damp phlegm
Black	Extreme cold or heat with deep penetration of body

INDEX FINGER VENULE (IFV)

Sign	Pattern
Indistinct, neither superficial nor deep, and red mixed with yellow	Normal
Red tinged with yellow, indistinct, and unexposed distal to Wind Pass	Normal
Easy to see, superficial, and exposed	Exterior
Difficult to see, deep, and indistinct	Interior
Shallow appearance	Light disease
Deep appearance	Serious condition
Venule visible in Wind Pass (first segment)	Mild, superficial EPI
Venule visible in Energy Pass (second segment)	Moves from exterior to interior, affects meridians
Venule visible in Vital Pass (third segment)	Critical internal organ invasion
Bright red	EPI (exterior)
Light red	Deficient and cold
Red	Excess heat
Deep red	Accumulated heat
Dull yellow	Spleen disharmony
Purplish or purplish red	Internal heat
Pale	Deficiency
Color remains after pressing	Excess
Irregular	Chronic
Narrow and fine	Abdominal pain
Bluish	Serious fright and pain
Blue-purple	Convulsions, pain, and blood stagnation
Cyanotic	Convulsions or pain
Cyanotic purple	Liver wind, heat dyspepsia from improper diet, phlegm obstruction of qi, fright, or pain
Black or purplish black	Serious, life-threatening stagnation of blood and collaterals
Bluish black	Life threatening
Floating	Superficial

COMPLEXION

Sign	Pattern
Blue	Liver
Red	Heart heat
Yellow	Spleen
White	Lung
Green	Liver wind or deficient stomach/spleen
Dark or black	Kidney
Blue face	Convulsions
Flushed face	Excess heat
Yellow face	Indigestion, impaired spleen, damp, weak constitution, or deficiency
White face	Cold and deficient
Dark face	Severe pain
Green-white	Cold (perverse yin)
Blue-green	Toxic wind heat
Yellow-red	Yang heat
Yellow with emaciation and with swollen, enlarged abdomen	Deficient stomach/spleen
Yellow and lusterless with white patches on face	Intestinal parasites
Yellow with yellow sclera	Jaundice
Blue-purple	Cold, pain, blood stagnation, or convulsions
Blue and pale with furrowed brow	Internal cold or abdominal pain
Blue-gray	Mental cloudiness or convulsions
Blue with purple lips and short breath	Qi and blood stagnation due to obstructed lung qi
Dim black	Congenital deficiency or cold accumulation and obstruction
Black or cyanotic Sauce Receptacle (CV 24)	Convulsions
Dark	Toxins
Intermittent fresh red flushing of cheeks	Excess yang due to deficient yin
Pale	Deficient and cold
Pale and puffy	Yang-deficiency edema (yin edema)
Suddenly grayish; pale, cold limbs; and perspiration	Yang qi collapse
Pale with pale lips	Blood deficiency
Pale with perspiration	Deficient lung qi and defensive qi
Pale and sallow complexion	Spleen deficiency
Glossy pale complexion	Qi deficiency
Pale complexion with pale red lips and fingernails	Blood deficiency

SIGN	PATTERN
Dreadfully pale complexion with cold extremities	Sudden collapse
Pale complexion and edema	Yang deficiency
Cyanotic complexion and lips	Serious liver wind, cold, or abdominal pain
Cyanotic complexion, twitch, fright, and palpitation	Convulsions
Cyanotic and tachypnea	Qi stagnation or blood stasis
Red with flushing	Fever
Local flushing of zygomatic regions in afternoon	Deficient yin fire
Fading sallow complexion	Deficient blood
Sallow and gloomy black complexion	Liver/kidney deficiency (critical)

FACE AREAS

SIGN	PATTERN
FOREHEAD	**HEART**
Red	Normal
Black	Abnormal
Bluish black	Convulsions, high fever, or abdominal pain
Yellowish	Deficient yin heat conditions
EYELIDS, LEFT CHEEK	**LIVER**
Blue	Normal
White	Abnormal
Red	Wind or fever
Bluish black	Convulsions, fever, or abdominal pain
Pale red	Onset of fever, coughing, or phlegm
RIGHT CHEEK, FRONTAL PROTUBERANCE	**LUNG**
White	Normal
Red	Abnormal
Striking red	Respiratory disease
EARLOBES, CHIN	**KIDNEY**
Red	Heat
NOSTRIL WINGS	**STOMACH**
BETWEEN nostrils and mouth corners	**SPLEEN**

MOUNTAIN BASE (SHAN GEN)

Sign	Pattern
Blue vein	Stomach/spleen deficiency
Bluish tint	Initial stage of stomach/spleen-deficiency pattern
Black	Kidney wind cold
Pale	Accumulated phlegm in lung
Cyanotic	Liver wind

EYES

Sign	Pattern
Dull and listless	Deficiency
Watering	Severe common cold or measles
Red sclera	Wind heat
Eyelid puffiness	Edema
Pink and gummy	Liver heat
Red eyelids and excess tears	Measles
Staring and hazy	Heat or malnutrition
Sunken eye sockets	Liver exhaustion
Sudden blindness	Yin and blood exhaustion
Staring with fixed gaze	Liver qi exhaustion
Pupil dilation	Stomach/spleen weakness
Dull, yellowish, or small pupils	Prolonged illness, difficult cure
Yellow sclera	Internal damp heat or spleen damp (jaundice)
Yellow and turbid sclera	Damp accumulation and stasis
Light blue sclera	Constitutional weakness and hyperactive liver
Black spots in sclera	Intestinal parasites
Dilated/shrunken pupils	Kidney qi exhaustion
Slight corneal opacity	Malnutrition
Murky and yellow with shrunken irises	Lingering and intractable condition
Red and eroded canthus	Retained damp heat in either intestine or both
White membrane encroaching on cornea	Malnutrition
Angry staring	Excessive liver qi
Pronounced pupil dilation	Stomach/spleen qi deficiency
Whites of eyes turning up	Stirring liver wind

NOSE

Sign	Pattern
Yellow	Normal
Red and dry	Heat
Runny	EPI
Thick mucus, or dry nostrils	Lung heat
Flaring nostrils, emphasized inhalation, shortness of breath, and profuse sweating	Lung exhaustion
Red	Deficient spleen yin heat
Bleeding	Accumulated heat in lung meridian
Trembling nostrils	Lung qi blockage or pneumonia
Dry nostrils	Lung heat or dryness
Stuffy, runny nose	Lung wind cold
Red with dry tip	Spleen heat
Deathly yellow	Spleen failure
Measles at tip	Complete exhibition and steady improvement

EARS

Sign	Pattern
Sensation of warmth or flushing at ears	Wind cold attack
Ear swelling and pain with discharge	Liver/gallbladder fire flaring upward
Diffused swelling around earlobe	Toxic wind heat invasion of gallbladder
Haggard and shriveled	Critical kidney water exhaustion
Cyanotic venules	Stirring liver wind

LIPS AND MOUTH

Sign	Pattern
Throat inflammation	Wind heat EPI
Red and swollen gums with erosion	Stomach fire flaring upward
Delayed teeth eruption	Kidney qi deficiency
Swollen tonsils	Retained heat in lung/stomach
Mouth ulcers	Accumulated heat in heart/spleen
White granules	Thrush
Pale lips	Spleen and blood deficiency

SIGN	PATTERN
Bright red lips	Heat pathogens
Cherry lips	Qi and yin damage
Scorched red lips	Depressed heat in heart and spleen
Cyanosis around lips	Liver invading spleen or convulsions
Cyanotic lips	Cold or blood stasis
Dry mouth and lips	Heat depleting fluids
Scorched purple or black lips	Blood heat damaging yin
Red, swollen, and painful lips	Spleen heat
Lip shrinkage	Spleen exhaustion
Drooling at mouth corners	Spleen cold
Grinding teeth in sleep	Stomach/spleen heat dyspepsia or parasites

FINGERNAILS

SIGN	PATTERN
Purplish	Heat
Red	Cold
Cyanotic	Heart pain
Black	Liver qi exhaustion
Pale and fragile	Blood deficiency
Purple or drumstick fingers	Qi stagnation, blood stasis, and deficient heart yang

Palpating
氣

Using palpation to assess a child differs slightly from using the process with adults. Because adults present a denser structure, palpation focuses primarily on pulses, points, and meridians. Children present a relatively more open and accessible body structure, so you can obtain information through direct palpation of the body.

Abdomen

With children, palpating the abdomen is usually substituted for pulse palpation. The abdomen is a significant indicator of many specific and general conditions. The smaller the child, the greater the proportion of the abdomen to the overall body. This presents a good opportunity to evaluate an easily accessible and understandable aspect of the child's condition: The abdomen is reflective of a major portion of energetic activity. Developing skill in abdominal assessment and treatment is vital to pediatric massage.

Skin

The skin reflects organ relationships to EPIs, fluid transformation, and temperature.

Body

Body palpation can provide valuable information regarding the effects of internal imbalances on structural integrity and development.

Pulses

Pulse diagnosis is not useful until the child reaches five to seven years of age. Even then you can use only one finger to palpate all three pulse positions. As the child grows, two, and then three fingers can be used for pulse taking. Less emphasis is put on pulse diagnosis in children than adults. As children grow, however, the pulse takes on more importance.

ABDOMEN	
SIGN	PATTERN
Soft, tender, and warm	Normal
Child prefers warmth	Cold
Child prefers cold	Heat
Soft with pain relieved by pressure	Deficiency and cold
Hard with pain aggravated by pressure	Excess heat
Hard with sharp pain	Excess
Distended with a shallow sensation upon pressure	Gas distension
Liquid sounds	Liquid accumulation
Tossing, shouting, or crying while holding abdomen	Abdominal pain
Tough, scorching abdomen	Accumulation and stagnation in either intestine or both
Abdominal distension with percussion sounds like drum	Stagnant qi

SKIN

Sign	Pattern
Hot with no perspiration	EPI invasion at surface
Cold with excessive perspiration	Deficient yang and defensive qi
Swollen skin that pits when pressed	Retained damp edema
Pitting that disappears when released	Pathogenic wind in lung impairing water regulation
Dry	Depleted fluids (dehydration from improper feeding, vomiting, or diarrhea)
Dry with impaired elasticity	Dehydration (qi and fluid consumption)
Relaxed muscles, loose skin, and fading yellow complexion	Deficient spleen qi
Scorching heat at palms and soles	Deficient yin or excess yang ming interior heat
Scorching heat in chest with short breath	Phlegm retention and lung heat
Tough, scorching abdomen	Accumulation and stagnation in either intestine or both

HEAD/NECK/BODY

Sign	Pattern
Slightly concave head with incomplete fontanel closure	Normal (below 18 months of age)
Headache, aversion to cold, and fever	Exterior
Abdominal pain, diarrhea, and cold limbs	Interior
Rubbing head and eyes	Headache or dizziness
Incomplete fontanel closure	Deficient kidney qi
Concave fontanel after vomiting and diarrhea	Deficient body fluids
Raised fontanel, high fever, and vomiting	Flaring heat and fire
Painful lymph nodules in neck	Phlegm toxins
Chronically cold limbs	Yang deficiency
Flaccid neck, slim physique, weak tendons and bones, wizened skin, emaciated calf, and crooked toes (with dull expression, shrinking lips, slobbery mouth, and sallow, sparse hair)	Congenital deficiency and/or nutritional imbalance
Enlarged head, shrinking jaw, widened anterior fontanel, and pupils turning downward	Delayed closure of fontanel
Crooked lower limbs, sparse hair, widened fontanels, and chest wall deformity	Rickets
Relaxed muscles, loose skin, and fading yellow complexion	Deficient spleen qi

SIGN	PATTERN
Sparse, withered, and sallow hair that falls out	Blood deficiency
Child sits upright, tachypnea with wheezing due to phlegm	Asthma
Tossing, shouting, or crying while holding abdomen	Abdominal pain
Neck stiffness, limb twitch, and opisthotonos	Convulsions
Child lies supine and listless without movement	Deficiency due to prolonged or serious illness

PULSES

SIGN	PATTERN
SUPERFICIAL	**EXTERIOR**
Forceful	Excess
Forceless	Deficiency or wind cold EPI
Slow	Wind cold
Rapid	Wind heat
Slippery	Wind phlegm
Slow and irregular	Damp wind
DEEP	**INTERIOR**
Forceful	Excess
Forceless	Deficiency or qi stagnation
Rapid	Heat
Slow	Cold
SLOW (LESS THAN 5 TO 6 PER BREATH)	**COLD**
Forceful	Excess, obstruction, or cold
Forceless	Deficiency or cold
Energetic	Cold or stagnation
Feeble	Deficient yang
RAPID (MORE THAN 8 PER BREATH)	**HEAT**
Forceful	Excess heat
Forceless	Deficiency yin heat
Superficial	Exterior heat
Deep	Interior heat
WIRY	**ABDOMINAL PAIN OR CONVULSIONS**
Rolling	Accumulated excess phlegm heat, or food retention

SIGN	PATTERN
WEAK AND FLOATING	QI AND BLOOD DEFICIENCY OR DAMP EPI INVASION
ENERGETIC	EXCESS
FEEBLE	DEFICIENT
DEFICIENT	QI AND BLOOD DEFICIENCY
REPLETE	EPI DOMINANCE OR HEALTHY QI DEFICIENCY
SLIPPERY	PHLEGM RETENTION, UNDIGESTED FOOD, OR EXCESS HEAT
STRINGY AND TAUT	LIVER, GALLBLADDER, PAIN, OR PHLEGM RETENTION
STRINGY AND RAPID	HEAT
STRINGY AND SLOW	COLD
IRREGULAR, INTERMITTENT, AND SLOW	YIN EXCESS, QI STAGNATION, OR BLOOD STASIS
IRREGULAR AND ABRUPT	YANG HYPERACTIVITY, HEAT, QI STAGNATION, BLOOD STASIS, PHLEGM RETENTION, OR UNDIGESTED FOOD

Listening and Smelling

Listening and smelling provide important information on a child's general condition as well as some specific patterns. Pediatric listening assessment includes voice/sounds and breath.

Voice and Sounds

The voice and sounds produced by a child can give you good supplementary information on the organs or location of the disharmony.

Breath

The quality of a child's breath can also provide information on which organ is involved and how serious the condition is.

VOICE AND SOUNDS

Sign	Pattern
Clear, loud speech	Normal
Untalkative and cold	Deficiency
Coughing, hoarse voice, productive mucus, and nasal obstruction	Wind cold EPI
Coughing, restrained voice, thick yellow mucus, and hard to expectorate	Retained heat in lung
Chronic cough and hoarse voice	Deficient lung qi
Coughing, hoarse voice, sounds like striking broken bamboo	Laryngitis or diphtheria
Dry cough	Lung dryness
Fluent cough with free phlegm discharge	Mild condition
Trembling sound	Spleen
Loud voice	Excess EPI
Giggling, flat speech	Heart
Loud groaning and touching chest	Stomach
Feeble crying and weak voice	Deficiency
Crying with tears	Excess
Crying without tears	Deficiency
Crying not alleviated by normal methods, on and off, shrill, unhurried then anxious	Abdominal pain
Crying with shaking head and heat	Head pain
Crying with refusing food and slobbering	Mouth ulcers
Muffled voice (strong then feeble)	Serious EPI
Muffled voice (feeble then strong)	Internal injury
Muffled voice and sneezing	External pathogen excess
Feeble voice and shortness of breath	Deficient ying qi
Feeble voice and low tones	Kidney qi deficiency
Shouting and scolding	Liver pain
Frowning and groaning	Headache
Groaning, shaking head, and touching cheeks	Toothache
Groaning and failing to stand	Low back pain
Difficult cough without discharge	Serious condition
Deep harsh cough and sticky yellow phlegm	Exogenous wind heat
Cough with clear loud sound and clear nasal discharge	Exogenous wind cold
Paroxysmal cough and whoops with inspiration	Whooping cough
Productive cough and dyspnea	Pulmonary disease
Cough with hoarse sound like barking	Diphtheria

SIGN	PATTERN
Incoherent babbling	Ying invasion by fire
Hoarse voice	Throat; vocal chord disorders; or internal accumulated wind, phlegm, and heat
Talkativeness and fever	Excess yang
Reluctant speech and coldness	Yin deficiency
Shrill shout	Severe pain
Coma or delirium	Invasion of pericardium by pathogens

BREATH

SIGN	PATTERN
Shortness of breath, then diaphragm distension	Lung
Diaphragm distension, then shortness of breath	Spleen
Deficient breath with trembling sound	Spleen
Shortness of breath, asthmatic breathing, nostril wing trembling, and gurgling in throat	Accumulated phlegm in lung
Asthmatic breathing, raised shoulders, dyspnea, restlessness, hoarse voice, and blue-purple complexion and lips	Critical throat obstruction due to sore throat
Feeble respiration and weeping vocal sounds when breathing	Lung qi collapse
Husky, forceful breathing	Excess EPI
Shortness of breath, productive cough, and dyspnea	Pulmonary disease
Feeble breath with sobbing sound during inspiration	Lung qi exhaustion

Inquiring
氣

Although the inquiring phase may be less productive with children than adults, you should still explore all related areas with the child and parent. Often a parent will think certain information is not relevant when in fact it may prove very useful to an accurate assessment. The inquiry phase may take longer with children, given the limitations of their communication skills and/or of the parent's memory.

It is possible to question even young children with simple terms, respect, and the expectations that they know themselves, and that good information may be produced. It is crucial to speak patiently with children and listen attentively. All too frequently adults can overpower children by talking too much. Good listening skills can produce good information in a difficult situation.

The pediatric inquiry assessment includes temperature, urine and stool, perspiration, diet, thirst, and behavior.

Temperature

Information on a child's temperature can provide you with important clues to the types and seriousness of EPIs.

Urine and Stool

Qualities of urine and stool are very strong indicators of stomach/spleen function and excess/deficiency and hot/cold syndromes.

Perspiration

The child's degree of perspiration also indicates stages of EPIs; it is also a general indication of yin/yang and qi/blood.

Diet

Information on diet provides important insight about the quality of the child's nourishment, the possible etiology of his or her condition, and the functioning of the stomach/spleen. It is reflective of the overall nature of the condition.

TEMPERATURE	
SIGN	PATTERN
Prefers cold	Heat
Prefers heat	Cold
Fever, chills, no or spontaneous sweating, and wind aversion	Wind cold EPI
Constant feverish body and palms	Deficient yin or internal injury
Fever, chills, and an absence of perspiration	Wind cold EPI
Fever, wind aversion, and perspiration	Wind heat EPI
Persistent fever and an absence of chills	Interior moving pathogenic heat

SIGN	PATTERN
Fever, huddling to keep warm, pale complexion, cold mouth, stuffy nose, nasal discharge, and sneezing	Exterior heat
Fever; hot mouth; deep-colored urine; constipation; and child desires drinks, exposes head, stretches limbs	Interior heat
Alternating chills and fever	Half-exterior, half-interior
Continuous, protracted fever without exterior syndromes, along with hot palms and soles	Interior damage or deficient yin
Summertime, protracted high fever, thirst, hyperhidrosis, and anuria	Summer heat
Yellow complexion, hot abdomen, and nocturnal fever	Overeating
Nocturnal fever and sour, fetid, undigested food in vomit or stool	Dyspepsia of milk
Nocturnal fever, drowsiness, abdominal fullness and distension, vomiting, and diarrhea	Dyspepsia of food
Nocturnal fever, diarrhea with greenish liquid, and fright crying	Dyspepsia or fright
Continuous nocturnal fever, emaciation, and enlarged head and abdomen	Malnutrition
Nocturnal fever, emaciation, cough, hemoptysis, vexation, and hot palms and soles	Deficient yin heat or consumptive syndrome
Feeble limbs, gray complexion, pale lips, spontaneous sweating, and slight aversion to cold	Yang deficiency
Chills and an absence of fever	Internal cold or deficient yang
Lassitude, glossy pale complexion, pale lips, spontaneous perspiration, and slight aversion to cold	Deficient yang or fever

URINE AND STOOL

SIGN	PATTERN
Yellow stool, neither too hard nor too moist	Normal
Clear, light yellow urine	Normal
Scanty deep-colored urine in hot weather	Normal
Light-colored urine in an infant with febrile disease	Condition improving
Loose stool or diarrhea	Deficiency
Frequent urination or enuresis	Vital qi deficiency
Frequent and loose stools	Spleen deficiency
Brown urine	Heat

SIGN	PATTERN
Deep red or brown urine	Hematuria
Turbid urine	Dyspepsia due to improper diet
Deep yellow-red urine	Damp heat
Yellow-red urine, oliguria, dysuria	Down-pouring damp heat
Clear urine, no odor	Cold, spleen/kidney deficiency, or deficient cold bladder
Dribbling urination with stabbing pain	Stranguria
Long passing of clear urine at night or enuresis	Kidney qi deficiency
Sticky and foul stool	Heat
Watery and foul stool	Cold
Constipation with heat signs	Yang stasis
Constipation with cold signs	Cold stasis
Watery diarrhea, foul mucous stools, burning anus, and heat signs	Excess heat
Brown diarrhea and scanty urine	Damp heat
Dry stool, or sheep droppings with several days of no stool	Excess heat in either intestine or both, yin deficiency, or fluid exhaustion
Loose stool with white milky masses or yellow stool with undigested food particles and spoiled-eggs odor	Stomach/spleen injured by excess feeding
Stool with mucus, blood, and tenesmus	Dysentery or damp heat in either intestine or both
Bloody, soy-sauce-colored stool in nursing infants with occasional crying	Obstruction in either intestine or both
Loose stool with fetid odor	Stagnant interior damp heat
Loose stool with coagulated masses	Dyspepsia due to improper diet
Incessant, watery diarrhea with undigested food	Spleen/kidney deficiency
Pale, watery, frothy diarrhea	Exogenous wind cold
Red or white and sticky, jellylike stool	Damp heat accumulation
Dark stool with crying fits	Obstruction in either intestine or both
Dry stool and constipation	Interior deficient yin heat
Sour, fetid, and loose stool	Improper feeding
Fetid stool	Blazing heat in either intestine or both
Clear, cold, and stenchy stool	Cold in either intestine or both
Constipation at early stage of condition	Excess heat in large intestine
Prolonged constipation	Depletion of body fluids
Clear, dilute, and rotten-fish stool	Cold
Dysentery with pus and blood in stool	Excess heat in large intestine
Watery diarrhea	Down-pouring water and damp

PERSPIRATION

SIGN	PATTERN
Slight forehead sweat while sleeping	Normal
No sweating, fever, or chill	Exterior, excess
Sweating, fever, and chill	Exterior, deficiency
Sweating, no chill, fever, and heat aversion	Interior
Lassitude with sweating upon exertion	Yang deficiency
Spontaneous daytime sweat upon slight exertion	Qi deficiency
Night sweats	Yin deficiency or qi and yin deficiency
Spontaneous, profuse daytime sweating	Deficient qi and weak defensive qi
Profuse, continuous sweating	Yang exhaustion (critical collapse)

DIET

SIGN	PATTERN
Stomachache relieved after eating	Deficiency
Stomachache worse after eating	Excess
Prefers hot food	Stomach cold and cold in either intestine or both
Prefers cold food	Stomach heat and heat in either intestine or both
Hunger but no appetite with stomach distress	Stomach phlegm or fire obstruction
Increased food intake, hunger, and weight loss	Flaming stomach fire
Good appetite with abdominal distension	Weak spleen with strong stomach
Abdominal distension after eating	Qi stagnation and indigestion
Poor appetite with abdominal fullness or distension	Excess food
Excessive eating and stools with emaciation	Hyperfunction of stomach/spleen (malnutrition)
Anorexia, constipation, and frequent belching	Food stagnation
Anorexia and concurrent diarrhea	Failure of spleen to transport
Excessive polyphagia, skinniness, and unusual eating addictions	Parasites

THIRST

Sign	Pattern
Extreme thirst, child prefers cold fluids	Interior heat
Profuse drinking	Yang pathogenic factors invading interior
Thirst without desire to drink	Genuine yin loss

BEHAVIOR

Sign	Pattern
Restless in day, quiet at night	Yang
Restless at night, quiet in day	Yin
Quiet behavior	Qi deficiency
Restless	Strong pathogenic factors

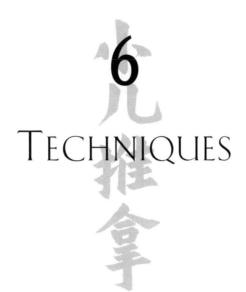

6
TECHNIQUES

AMONG THE DISTINGUISHING CHARACTERISTICS of tui na are its number and intricacies of hand techniques relative to other types of massage. This may also help explain why there are few skilled tui na practitioners in the West. While some of the hand movements are simple and similar to those of other massage styles, others are unique and require precision, dexterity, and grace. The difference between a "massage" technique and a tui na manipulation is that the latter is specifically focused toward influencing the energetic and physical structures of the body. This may seem like a fine distinction, but it is just this subtlety that separates tui na from other types of physical manipulation.

Chinese pediatric massage involves numerous techniques, both basic and complex. Much can be accomplished by the proficient use of several basic techniques. However, like a dancer, the more skill and grace you can bring to your performance through a variety of techniques, the more you can achieve during a treatment.

Touch
氣

Massage is about touch. The quality of touch, depth of pressure, and overall gentleness of the technique are important considerations. Remember that children's energy is easily accessible, and massage does not require heavy pressure to be effective. With adults you may need to use pressure to achieve the desired results; this is not the case with children.

While it is difficult to describe the proper degree of touch in words, a general guideline is to limit pressure to the skin level. Do not try to press deeply into the muscles. With light pressure you will be able to perform the movement of the technique very quickly and briskly. *Light, quick,* and *brisk* are the key words when you are performing these techniques. Books and videos can be useful aids in this learning process; however, seek feedback whenever possible from a trained practitioner.

Technique Qualities

The four requirements of a good technique are duration, force, gentleness, and rhythm (evenness). These are the minimum standards to produce the desired effect from the technique.

Duration

The technique must be done at a high level of proficiency for a long enough time to achieve the desired effect. Performing a motion properly for two minutes and then lapsing into poor technique is not sufficient.

Force

The technique must achieve enough power to deal with the energetic condition of the child. Force does not mean pressure or physical strength. The force of a technique is the energetic power that results from the appropriate hand motion.

Gentleness

The technique should not create any more pain than the child is already experiencing. Each technique should be performed in a manner that is efficient and effective, yet also takes into account the child's tolerance level.

Rhythm or Evenness

This is the smooth, regular, continuous pattern of applying the technique to the point. Of the four requirements, rhythm may be the most difficult to master. Each technique has its own rhythm. It is a very subjective quality, difficult to describe through words.

However, rhythm is very comfortable and smooth when it is present and very conspicuous by its absence.

It is impossible to teach good technique in a book; you must have guidance by a qualified practitioner. I present the information here as a reminder to students as well as a guide for practitioners who already have some skill at hand manipulations.

Tonification and Clearing

Tonification is used to supplement a deficiency; to strengthen an aspect that is weak. Clearing is used to decrease an excessive or stagnant energetic condition. This is an important distinction in all of Chinese medicine, but especially so with children. Because their energetic nature is relatively unstable, children can be easily influenced by these techniques.

You can achieve tonification and clearing through your choice of technique and of manipulation quality. Some techniques (such as chafe) are inherently tonifying; others (such as push apart) are inherently clearing. The qualities of tonifying techniques include light force, slow speed, and long duration. Clearing techniques are performed with strong force, quick speed, and short duration.

Your choice of tonification or clearing is an ongoing clinical process. It is important not to develop a routine of using the same technique and qualities. Children vary considerably; even in one individual, the course of an illness can change quickly. Always assess and reevaluate your choice of technique to fit the moment. Remember that an accurate assessment is crucial to the selection of the appropriate technique—and sometimes of technique quality.

In China tui na techniques are perfected on a rice bag before being practiced on a patient. Depending on the technique, it may take many hours of practice before you attain proficiency. The rice bag is a good method for training and should be adopted by any serious student. See appendix A; Technique Practice on a Rice Bag.

Massage techniques are divided into single and multiple techniques. Single techniques are basic repetitions of the same movement on a point. In this chapter I will describe single techniques in a general manner. The specific movement of the technique will depend on the selected point.

Multiple techniques are more complex, requiring the performance of several manipulations simultaneously or in sequence. You should be very competent with all single techniques before you try to incorporate multiple techniques into your protocols.

Single Techniques
氣

Press Techniques

This group of techniques involves the application of simple pressure held stationary on the selected point.

PRESS

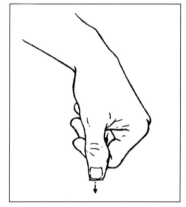

PRESS

Technique: Use your thumb, middle finger, or palm to press the point. Gradually increase the pressure from light to heavy. The depth and force depend on the condition. After forceful pressure, follow with press rotate.

Action: Warm meridians, clear collaterals, tranquilize mind, relieve pain.

PRESS ROTATE

Technique: This technique starts with a press and then adds a rotary movement with the part of the hand listed below. Move your hand and wrist from your elbow in a relaxed, rhythmic, and swaying motion. The part of your hand in contact with the point should remain stationary. Your forearm describes a tight spiraling motion

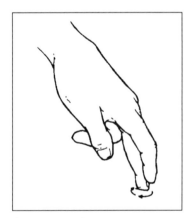

PRESS ROTATE: *1 FINGER*

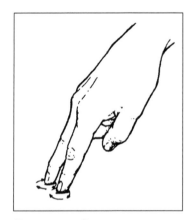

PRESS ROTATE: *2 FINGERS*

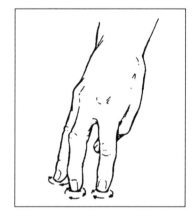

PRESS ROTATE: *3 FINGERS*

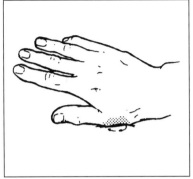

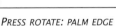

PRESS ROTATE: PALM EDGE

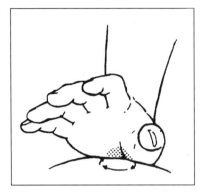

PRESS ROTATE: LOWER PALM

that travels down to the point in a funnel-like shape. The movement should be even, soft, and rhythmic, bringing the skin along with the movement of your hand.

Action: Drive qi, activate blood, clear meridians, harmonize collaterals, open organ obstructions.

Fingers (1, 2, 3): Using one, two, or three fingers (depending on the point), begin with a press and gradually begin the press rotate rotary motion, focusing on your fingertips or pads.

Palm edge: Use your greater thenar eminence as the only point of contact with the point. Your hand and wrist will be slightly angled to achieve this position. The rotary motion mainly comes from a loose, flexible wrist.

Lower palm: Use the center of the lowest aspect of your palm. This requires less wrist action and more movement from your forearm and shoulder.

FINGERNAIL PRESS

Technique: Use a thumbnail to apply force gradually and penetratingly. Do not cut the skin. Afterward, apply press rotate to relieve pain.

Action: Calm fright, sober mind, open passes, dredge orifices, quell spasms, relieve twitch.

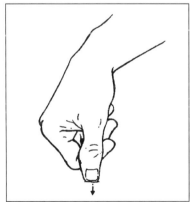

FINGERNAIL PRESS

Push Techniques

In push techniques you use your individual fingers; some combination of your thumb, index, and middle fingers; or the edge of your palm to push forcefully in a specific direction relative to the point. Your technique should be light and rapid, but it should not irritate the skin.

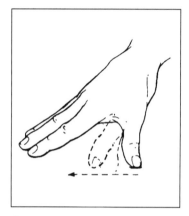

PUSH: THUMB

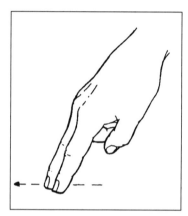

PUSH: INDEX FINGER

PUSH

Technique: Perform the push technique in a linear direction along the intended point (line) to avoid other points or meridians.

Action: Relax tendons, activate blood, clear meridians, relieve pain.

CHAFE

Technique: Using the ulnar aspect—not the edge— of your palm, perform a brisk, repetitive, back-and-forth movement. You should use very little force or pressure, although the chafe must be performed rapidly to produce the desired effect.

Action: Warm and clear meridians and collaterals, tonify deficiency, invigorate original yang.

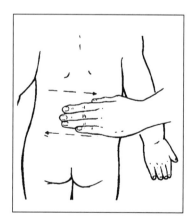

CHAFE

ROTATE PUSH

Technique: This technique is similar to press rotate except that the contact point of your hand does not stay stationary; it moves along the skin surface. Depending on the selected point, rotate in a circular motion according to the size of the point and the condition. Your fingers and hand should be relaxed and should conform to the shape of the body area. A flexible and loose wrist is important to maintain a smooth, rhythmic action. The direction of rotation depends on the condition.

Action: Regulate qi, harmonize blood, clear collaterals.

Index and middle fingers: Use the pads of your index and middle fingers to rotate in a circular motion over a small point area.

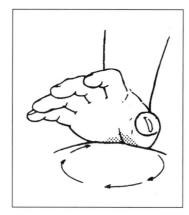

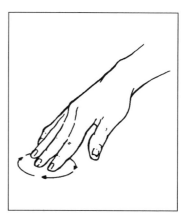

ROTATE PUSH: INDEX AND MIDDLE FINGERS

ROTATE PUSH: INDEX, MIDDLE, AND RING FINGERS

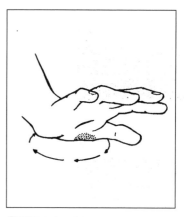

ROTATE PUSH: LOWER PALM

ROTATE PUSH: GREATER THENAR EMINENCE

Index, middle, and ring fingers: Use the pads of these fingers to rotate in a circular motion over the point area.

Lower center palm: Use your lesser thenar eminence or the center of your lower palm to make a circular rotation. Wrist action should accomplish the motion.

Greater thenar eminence: Use the large, fleshy aspect of your greater thenar eminence to contact the point. A loose wrist at a small angle should accomplish a rotational motion on the point.

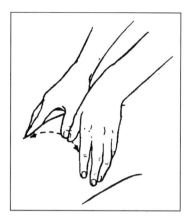

PUSH APART

PUSH APART

Technique: Using the tips of both thumb pads or your greater thenar eminence, push from the center of the point, moving both hands simultaneously away toward the periphery. The movement is one-directional and rapid with light pressure. The size and region of the point will determine the specifics of your motion.

Action: Regulate and harmonize yin/yang, drive qi, activate blood, separate clear from turbid, drain turbid.

PUSH CONVERGE

Technique: This technique is similar to push apart (above) except that the direction of movement is from the periphery to the center. Using the tips of both thumbs or your greater thenar eminence, push from the periphery to the center of the point.

Action: Regulate and harmonize yin/yang, drive qi, activate blood.

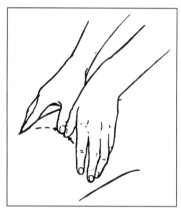

PUSH CONVERGE

SPINAL PINCH PULL

Technique: Begin at the sacrum with one hand on each side of the spine. Grip the skin with both of your thumbs and index fingers. Gently lift up and begin moving along the spine, continuously rolling the skin up and lifting it away from the spine. Continue along the length of the spine to C-7. This technique is only used in one direction, from inferior to superior.

Action: Regulate yin/yang, qi, blood; harmonize organs; promote smooth meridian function; tonify deficiency.

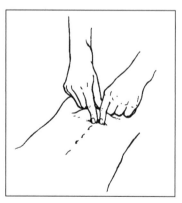

SPINAL PINCH PULL

GRASP

Technique: Using your thumb and index finger, gently grip the skin on the point, lifting quickly and repeatedly until the point begins to color.

Action: Induce perspiration, relieve exterior, clear orifices, sober mind, regulate and harmonize qi and blood.

RUB

Technique: Using your palm or index, middle, and ring finger pads, gently and slowly rub the point.

Action: Harmonize middle burner, rectify qi.

RUB ROLL

Technique: Hold the body part with both of your palms at opposite sides. Press your palms together and energetically rub-roll them back and forth, rapidly and rhythmically. Try to move your hands slowly yet still produce brisk movement of the body part.

Action: Regulate qi, harmonize blood, relax tendons and vessels.

POUND

Technique: Tap the point with your fingertip or the middle knuckle of a finger. The movement should be light, steady, and rhythmic.

Action: Calm fright, tranquilize mind, relax spasms.

PINCH SQUEEZE

Technique: Using both of your thumbs and index fingers, pinch and squeeze toward the point from four directions rapidly and repeatedly until sufficient coloring appears in the point.

Action: Resolve stasis, disperse accumulation, relax tendons, harmonize blood.

SHAKE

Technique: Hold the ends of the bones that form the affected joint. Rock circularly, swaying back and forth, increasing your range of motion and rate appropriately to the condition. Move gently, slowly, and rhythmically.

Action: Harmonize qi and blood, clear meridians and collaterals, facilitate joints.

RANGE OF MOTION

Technique: This technique depends on the movement potential of the body part in question. Each joint or area will move in its own particular way. Hold the area so as to facilitate the full spectrum of movement that it can naturally perform. Begin with slow, gentle, circular motions. Increase your pace, maintaining a gentle, rhythmic motion, then gradually wind down to a slow ending.

Action: Open and clear meridians and collaterals, drive qi, harmonize qi and blood.

RUB PALMS TOGETHER

Technique: Briskly rub your palms together, using little pressure but rapid, repetitive, back-and-forth motions. After generating significant heat (qi), approximately fifteen to twenty seconds, cover the point.

Action: Tonify deficiency, warm meridians and collaterals, nourish original yang.

Multiple Techniques
氣

BLACK DRAGON WAGS TAIL

Location: The elbow and little finger.

Technique: Hold the elbow and little finger; rock 20–30 times.

Action: Open blockages and obstructions, facilitate urination, relax bowels.

BLUE DRAGON WAGS TAIL

Location: Hand and elbow, Lesser Sea.

Technique: Support by holding Lesser Sea. Grasp four fingers and sway right and left 20–30 times.

Action: Reduce fever, relax bowels, relieve chest.

LASH HORSE TO CROSS GALAXY

Location: From the center of the palm to Vast Pool.

Technique: Press rotate Inner Palace of Labor, then push to Vast Pool, distal to proximal, 10–20 times *or* grasp (quickly) then release along the length of the point 10–20 times.

Action: Clear meridians, drive qi, facilitate joints.

MONKEY PLUCKS APPLES

Location: Bilateral ear tips and lobes.

Technique: Grip and lift the ear tips upward 10–20 times, then pinch and pull the earlobes downward 10–20 times.

Action: Drive qi, resolve phlegm, calm fright, tonify spleen and stomach.

OLD MAN PULLS THE FISH NET

Location: Thumb.

Technique: Fingernail press, and pinch Spleen Meridian; rock 20–40 times.

Action: Tonify spleen, promote digestion.

PHOENIX FLAPS WINGS

Location: Elbow to wrist.

Technique: Supporting the elbow, press, and fingernail press the depression before the lowest end of the radius and ulna; then rock the forearm right to left 20–30 times.

Action: Eliminate phlegm, sober mind, regulate and harmonize qi and blood.

PHOENIX SPREADS ONE WING

Location: Wrist and palm.

Technique: Grasp, and pinch Inner Palace of Labor and Outer Palace of Labor with one hand, rocking the child's hand with your other.

Action: Smooth qi flow, harmonize blood, warm meridians, tonify deficiency.

PHOENIX SPREADS WINGS

Location: Wrist and dorsal hand.

Technique: Fingernail press Vim Tranquillity and Imposing Agility while rocking the wrist upward and downward 20–50 times.

Action: Warm lung meridian, relieve dyspnea and distension, calm fright and palpitation, eliminate dysphagia.

PRESS ROTATE SPIRIT GATE, TORTOISE TAIL, AND BONE OF SEVEN SEGMENTS

Location: Navel, coccyx to L-2

Technique: Press rotate Spirit Gate and Tortoise Tail simultaneously. Push Bone of Seven Segments (upward to tonify, downward to clear) 40–80 times.

Action: *Tonify:* Stop diarrhea and dysentery. *Clear:* Clear damp heat of large intestine.

PRESS SHOULDER WELL

Location: Index and ring fingers, and shoulder.

Technique: Press, and fingernail press Shoulder Well with your middle finger, then grasp index and ring fingers and stretch, then whirl and rock 20–30 times.

Action: Promote qi circulation throughout body; a good technique with which to end a treatment.

RED PHOENIX NODS HEAD

Location: Middle finger and elbow.

Technique: Holding the elbow and grasping the middle finger, rock upward and downward.

Action: Open passes, smooth qi flow, nourish blood, tranquilize mind.

RED PHOENIX WAGS TAIL

Location: Inner Palace of Labor, Outer Palace of Labor, middle fingertip.

Technique: Fingernail press Outer Palace of Labor and Inner Palace of Labor with the thumb and index finger of one hand while you fingernail press the middle fingertip with your nail and rock 10–20 times.

Action: Harmonize qi and blood, calm fright.

ROCK LESSER SEA

Location: Hand, Lesser Sea, elbow joint.

Technique: Holding the elbow and Lesser Sea, cross the child's Tiger's Mouth with your own Tiger's Mouth and press Small Celestial Center; crook your hand and rock the forearm upward and downward 20–30 times.

Action: Smooth qi flow, generate blood, clear meridians, activate collaterals.

RUB AND RUB ROLL ALONG STRING

Location: Below Ribs to Abdominal Corner.

Technique: Have a second person hold the child while your five fingers roll and round rub both flanks from Below Ribs to Abdominal Corner 50–100 times, pressing the skin closely as if you were pressing a string.

Action: Smooth qi flow, resolve phlegm, eliminate chest oppression, dredge and disperse stagnation and accumulation.

ROTATING EAR AND ROCKING HEAD

Location: Both earlobes and head.

Technique: Twist and press the bilateral earlobes strenuously 20–30 times; then hold the head in both hands and rock left and right 10–20 times.

Action: Calm fright, harmonize qi and blood.

SOLITARY WILD GOOSE HOVERS ABOUT

Location: Forearm, palm, and thumb.

Technique: Push Spleen Meridian, Three Passes, Six Hollow Bowels, and Inner Palace of Labor. Repeat 10–20 times.

Action: Harmonize qi and blood, eliminate swelling and distension.

SWIFT-SHIFTING PRESS

Location: Pool at the Bend to the fingertips.

Technique: Press Pool at the Bend with four fingers and shift distally to Chief Tendon. Repeat 3–4 times. Then grip Yin Pool and Yang Marsh, bending four fingers upward and downward successively 20–50 times.

Action: Activate qi, clear lungs, resolve phlegm.

TIGER SWALLOWS A PREY

Location: Subservient Visitor, Kun Lun Mountains.

Technique: Snap your fingers at Subservient Visitor and Kun Lun Mountains (protected by a cloth).

Action: This first-aid technique helps regain consciousness, open orifices, sober mind, calm fright.

TWO DRAGONS PLAY WITH A PEARL

Location: Medial forearm.

Technique: With your index and middle fingers press Chief Tendon to Pool at the Bend (i.e., distal to proximal).

Action: Regulate qi, harmonize blood, calm fright.

TWO PHOENIXES SPREAD THEIR WINGS

Location: Both ears, head, and face.

Technique: Grip the bilateral ears with your index and middle fingers, lifting repeatedly several times. Then press, and fingernail press 10–20 times each: Hall of Authority, Great Yang, Auditory Convergence, Jawbone, Human Center, Sauce Receptacle.

Action: Expel wind cold, warm lung meridian.

WASPS GO OUT FROM CAVES

Location: Internal Palace of Labor, Inner Pass, Water (Inner Eight Symbols), Fire Palace.

Technique: Fingernail press Inner Palace of Labor and Chief Tendon. Push apart Large Transverse Line. Pinch squeeze Chief Tendon to Inner Pass. Finally, fingernail press Water Palace and Fire Palace 15–30 times.

Action: Promote diaphoresis, relieve exterior.

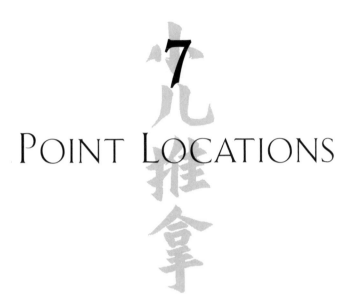

7

POINT LOCATIONS

MOST PRACTITIONERS OF ORIENTAL MEDICINE have an extensive familiarity with adult acupoints. In the case of pediatrics the definition and manipulation of points assume sightly different forms.

In general a *point* refers to a place where qi gathers and can be influenced. This is a fairly broad definition and does not necessarily imply constraints around location, size, and so on. For the purposes of pediatric massage, points are better defined as areas, rather than small dots; many points do not have the size or shape of a dot. For acupuncturists accustomed to inserting needles or massage practitioners applying finger pressure, this distinction is important. For example, the point Three Passes is a line located on the radial side of the medial forearm, running from the styloid process to the elbow transverse crease.

As I discussed in chapter 4, the development of the meridian and point systems is not mature at birth; it develops continuously through childhood. Over the centuries Chinese pediatricians have collected and categorized pediatric points based on their clinical experience. Thus, there has evolved a distinct set of pediatric points.

Some pediatric massage points are similar to adult acupoints, but others are unique to pediatrics. Moreover, pediatric points that have an adult acupoint counterpart should be defined and used according to the pediatric point definition. In some instances point names and locations are similar in children and adults; however, the energetic function may differ. For practitioners who treat only adults, this requires a certain shift in attitude and approach to points when treating children.

Pediatric points have never been Westernized by substituting a number for the Chinese name. In this book I have used English translations of the Chinese names to encourage you to become familiar with the *character* of the point, which is generally reflected in its name. Pin yin transliteration is not used, because most practitioners are not fluent in Chinese; it would create one more obstacle to understanding the nature of the point. For readers fluent in Chinese, however, I have given pin yin transliterations and acupuncture numbers for each point name after the English translation. See also appendix D, Point Names.

Even the most experienced practitioner will want to review the following points to gain a fresh perspective of their use in the treatment of children.

Hand Region

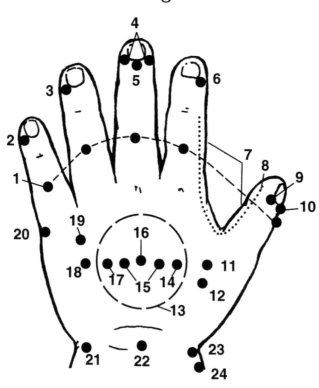

DORSAL HAND-POINT NAMES

20	Back Ravine	10	Lesser Metal Sound	12	Sweet Load
24	Broken Sequence	9	Maternal Cheek	4	Symmetric Upright
8	Celestial Gate to Tiger's Mouth	6	Metal Sound	7	Tiger's Mouth
19	Central Islet	21	Nursing the Aged	17	Two Horses
16	External Palace of Labor	5	Old Dragon	15	Two Leaf Door
1	Five Digital Joints	22	One Nestful Wind	11	Union Valley
14	Imposing Agility	13	Outer Eight Symbols	18	Vim Tranquillity
2	Lesser Marsh	3	Passage Hub	23	Yang Marsh

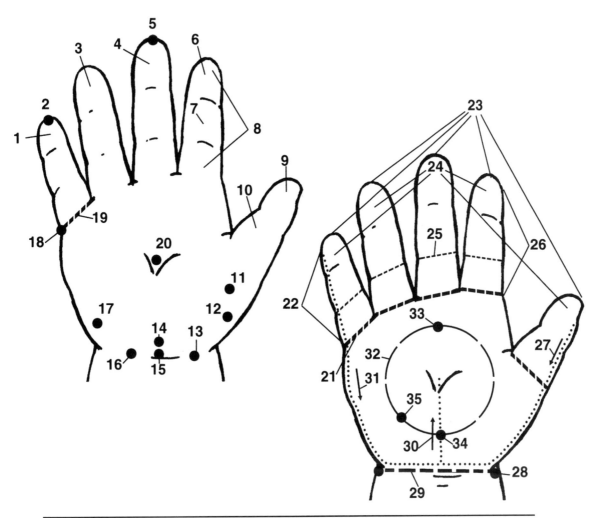

PALM HAND-POINT NAMES

13 Blue Tendon	20 Inner Palace of Labor	28 Snail Shell
5 Central Hub	19 Kidney Line	9 Spleen Meridian
15 Chief Tendon	1 Kidney Meridian	10 Stomach Meridian
33 Fire Palace (Inner Eight Symbols)	2 Kidney Summit	23 Ten Kings
12 Fish Border	26 Large Intestine Meridian	8 Three Digital Passes
30 Fish for Moon Under Water	29 Large Transverse Line	27 Transport Earth to Water
24 Five Meridians	6 Liver Meridian	31 Transport Water to Earth
25 Four Transverse Lines	3 Lung Meridian	34 Water (Inner Eight
7 Gallbladder Meridian	18 Palmar Small Transverse Line	Symbols)
35 Hand Celestial Gate	14 Small Celestial Center	16 White Tendon
4 Heart Meridian	22 Small Intestine Meridian	11 Wood Gate
32 Inner Eight Symbols	21 Small Transverse Lines	17 Yin Pool

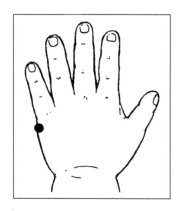

BACK RAVINE   HOU XI   SI 3

Location: Depression at the ulnar end of the palmar transverse crease (the junction between red and white skin, proximal to fifth metacarpal joint).

Technique: Fingernail press 20–40 times.

Action: Clear and invigorate kidney, promote urination.

Indications: Dysuria, dark urine.

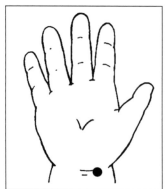

BLUE TENDON   QING JIN

Location: On the palmar transverse wrist crease, midway between Chief Tendon (midpoint) and Yang Marsh (radial end).

Technique: Press rotate 20–40 times, *or* fingernail press 3–5 times.

Action: Clear pericardium heat, improve eyesight.

Indications: Conjunctivitis, blurred vision.

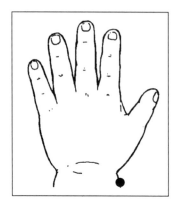

BROKEN SEQUENCE   LIE QUE   LU 7

Location: 1.5 cun superior to the wrist transverse crease, above the radial styloid process.

Technique: Grasp 5–10 times, *or* fingernail press 5–10 times.

Action: Ease mind, calm fright, induce perspiration, relieve exterior, refresh brain, depress adverse rising qi.

Indications: Convulsions, common cold with no perspiration, headache, dizziness, coma, deviation of eye and mouth, clenched teeth.

CELESTIAL GATE TO TIGER'S MOUTH   TIAN MEN RU HU KOU

Location: On the thumb, moving from its tip along the ulnar side (lateral edge) to the web.

Technique: Push distal to proximal 100–300 times, then press rotate Wood Gate 30–60 times.

Action: Smooth qi flow, harmonize blood circulation, warm meridians, disperse cold, stop vomiting and diarrhea, promote digestion, calm patient.

Indications: Anhidrosis, clenched teeth, sore throat, chest fullness.

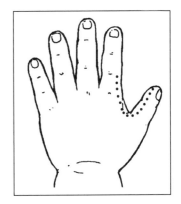

CENTRAL HUB   ZHONG CHONG   P 9

Location: Middle finger, center of the tip.

Technique: Fingernail press deeply 5–10 times, then press rotate 10–20 times.

Action: Induce perspiration, reduce fever, ease mind, calm fright, relieve spasms.

Indications: Cold aversion, hot body without perspiration, vexation, oppression, hectic fever, hot soles or palms, acute or chronic convulsions, thrush, swollen tongue.

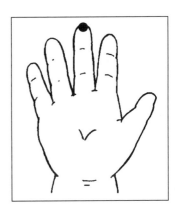

CENTRAL ISLET   ZHONG ZHU   TW 3

Location: With clenched fist, the dorsal hand between the fourth and fifth metacarpals, in the depression proximal to the metacarpophalangeal joint.

Technique: Press Rotate 100–300 times, *or* fingernail press 10–20 times.

Action: Expel wind heat.

Indications: Febrile diseases.

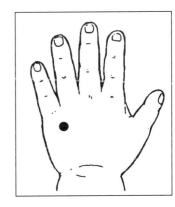

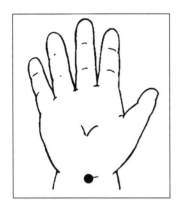

CHIEF TENDON   ZHONG JIN

Location: Midpoint on the palmar wrist transverse crease.

Technique: Press rotate 100–300 times, *or* fingernail press 3–5 times.

Action: Disperse heat, relieve spasms, ease mind, calm fright, reduce fever, disperse stagnation.

Indications: Convulsions, mental stress, diarrhea, vomiting, mouth ulcers, night crying, fever, toothache.

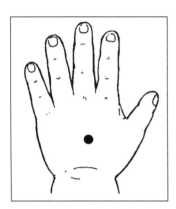

EXTERNAL PALACE OF LABOR   WAI LAO GONG

Location: Center of the dorsal hand (opposite Inner Palace of Labor).

Technique: Rotate push 100–200 times; *or* fingernail press 3–5 times, then rotate press 100–300 times.

Action: Warm yang, disperse pathologic cold, consolidate and warm lower burner, disperse external heat, promote digestion, remove stagnation, relieve pain.

Indications: Stool with undigested food, borborygmus, diarrhea, dysentery (cold), abdominal pain, hernia, prolapsed anus, intestinal parasites, exogenous diseases, enuresis, abdominal distension, hectic fever, hot body, headache.

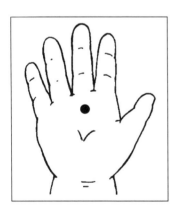

FIRE PALACE (INNER EIGHT SYMBOLS)   LI GONG

Location: On the palm, the twelve o'clock point in Inner Eight Symbols (see page 62.)

Technique: Push 100–200 times, *or* fingernail press 10–20 times.

Action: Clear excess heat.

Indications: Excess heat due to external pathogenic influences.

FISH BORDER   YU JI   LU 10

Location: On the greater thenar eminence, at the radial aspect of the first metacarpal bone (at the junction of red and white skin).

Technique: Fingernail press 5–10 times, then press rotate 20–40 times.

Action: Calm fright, eliminate abdominal distension, promote digestion, remove stagnation.

Indications: Convulsions, opisthotonos, abdominal distension or oppression.

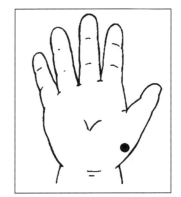

FISH FOR MOON UNDER WATER   SHUI DI LAO YUE

Location: Lateral border of the little fingertip, moving to Small Celestial Center then to Inner Palace of Labor.

Technique: Push 100–500 times.

Action: Clear pathological heat.

Indications: All heat patterns, especially those involving the heart.

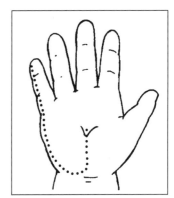

FIVE DIGITAL JOINTS   WU ZHI JIE

Location: Dorsal middle joint on each of the five fingers.

Technique: Press 3–5 times; *or* press rotate 100–200 times; *or* fingernail press 3–5 times, then press rotate 100–300 times.

Action: Resuscitate from unconsciousness, stop convulsions, open orifices, resolve phlegm, disperse cold and heat, disperse external pathogens, resolve phlegm.

Indications: Convulsions, spasms, coma, cough, runny nose, poor appetite, exogenous symptoms.

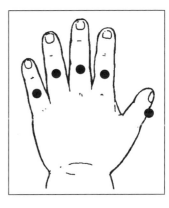

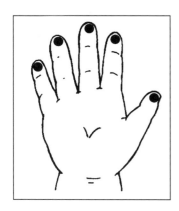

FIVE MERIDIANS   WU JING

Location: On the palmar side, the distal segments of all five fingers.

Technique: Rotate push 50–100 times, *or* push 50–100 times, *or* fingernail press 5–10 times, *or* press rotate 20–30 times.

Action: Tonify spleen, eliminate dampness, promote digestion, remove stagnation, expel wind, harmonize five zang organs.

Indications: Fever, chest oppression, abdominal distension, diarrhea, limb twitching.

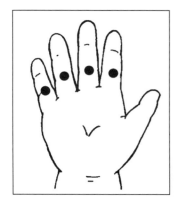

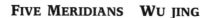

FOUR TRANSVERSE LINES   SUI WEN   X 25

Location: On the palmar aspect of the hand, the transverse lines at the second segment of all four fingers.

Technique: Fingernail press 3–5 times, then press rotate 30–50 times; *or* push back and forth 300–400 times.

Action: Relieve chest, facilitate diaphragm, promote digestion, resolve phlegm.

Indications: Abdominal distension, chest fullness or oppression, dyspnea, productive cough, chapped lips, abdominal pain, poor appetite.

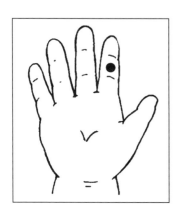

GALLBLADDER MERIDIAN   DAN JING   GB

Location: Index finger, palmar side of the second phalange.

Technique: *Clear:* Push distal to proximal 100–500 times. *Tonify:* Press rotate 100–500 times.

Action: Pacify and relax gallbladder, disperse gallbladder heat.

Indications: Earache, gallbladder meridian inflammation.

HAND CELESTIAL GATE   SHOU TIAN MEN

Location: On Inner Eight Symbols, the left palm at the four o'clock position, and the right palm at the eight o'clock position (see page 62).

Technique: Push from thumbtip to Hand Celestial Gate 30–60 times, *or* grasp Hand Celestial Gate and rock Lesser Sea 5–10 times.

Action: Drive qi, harmonize blood, promote digestion, relieve dyspepsia.

Indications: Disharmony of qi and blood, indigestion, stagnant food, vomiting, diarrhea.

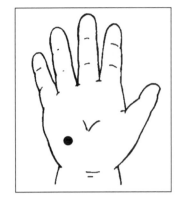

HEART MERIDIAN   XIN JING   H

Location: Middle finger, palmar pad of the distal phalange.

Technique:* *Tonify:* Press rotate 100–500 times. *Clear:* Push proximal to distal 100–500 times.

Action: Clear heat, calm fright.

Indications: High fever, coma, dark and scant urine, eruptions on mouth and tongue, dysuria, vexation, hot soles and palms, chest oppression, thrush.

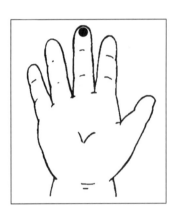

IMPOSING AGILITY   WEI LING

Location: Dorsal hand, between the second and third metacarpals (radial side of Outer Palace of Labor).

Technique: Press 3–5 times, then press rotate 30–50 times; *or* fingernail press 3–5 times, then press rotate 100–300 times.

Action: Resuscitate from coma, tranquilize mind, stop fainting, expel cold from extremities, stop convulsions.

Indications: Tinnitus, headache, convulsive unconsciousness, sudden fainting.

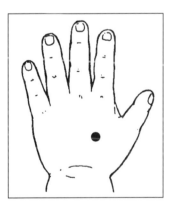

---

* Clinically, Heart Meridian is usually not directly manipulated. Heat issues can be reduced by pushing Water of Galaxy. Tonification can be accomplished by press rotating Spleen Meridian. An exception is extreme heart heat, which may be directly cleared.

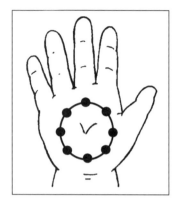

INNER EIGHT SYMBOLS

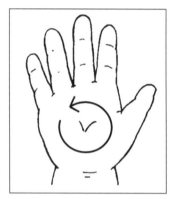

NORMAL FLOW (RIGHT HAND)

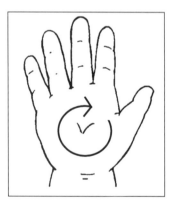

COUNTERFLOW (RIGHT HAND)

INNER EIGHT SYMBOLS   NEI BA GUA

Location: A circle 1 cun in radius around the midpoint of the palm (Inner Palace of Labor).

The Inner Eight Symbols refer to the Chinese Ba Gua. The eight symbols each refer to a particular element within nature that can be manipulated for a specific effect.

For those familiar with the *I Ching*, or the Ba Gua, the element locations can be described using the analogy of a clock face. Look at the left palm and imagine the Inner Eight Symbol circle there. At the junction of the third finger and the palm is twelve o'clock. Sky (Qian) is at four o'clock; Water (Kan) at six o'clock; Mountain (Gen) at eight o'clock; Thunder (Zhen) at nine o'clock; Wind (Xun) at ten o'clock; Fire (Li) at twelve o'clock; Earth (Kun) at two o'clock; and Ocean (Dui) at 3 o'clock.

The right-palm clock numbers are in reverse order; twelve and six o'clock are the same.

Technique: Rotate push 100–500 times.

The direction of rotation around Inner Eight Symbols is important. There are two directions of movement: normal flow and counterflow. In normal flow move clockwise around the child's left hand, counterclockwise around the right hand. In counterflow move counterclockwise around the child's left hand, clockwise around the right hand.

The action of normal flow is to raise qi, meaning to move it upward in the body. This is the typical tonifying action for children. However, some conditions are already moving upward in the body and would be aggravated by more upward movement. For example, coughing and vomiting are characterized by upward movement. For these types of conditions you should push Inner Eight Symbols in the counterflow direction. The action of counterflow is to descend qi in the body.

Action: Regulate and remove obstruction of qi and blood, harmonize five zang organs, relieve chest, resolve phlegm, facilitate diaphragm, promote digestion, depress adverse rising stomach qi. *Normal flow:* Raise qi. *Counterflow:* Descend qi.

Indications: Cough, diarrhea, abdominal distension, food stagnancy, vomiting, dyspnea (phlegm), dyspepsia, abdominal distension, anorexia, chest oppression, vexation, restlessness.

INNER PALACE OF LABOR   NEI LAO GONG   P 8

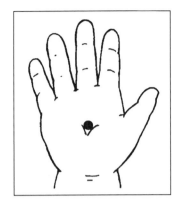

Location: Center of the palm; a flexed index or middle finger will touch the point.

Technique: Press rotate 50–300 times, *or* rotate push 30–100 times, *or* pound 50–300 times.

Action: Clear heat, relieve exterior symptoms, stop convulsions.

Indications: Fright, convulsions, common-cold fever, excess-heat syndromes, deficient yin heat syndromes, heart fever, vexation, internal heat, thrush, gum erosion, high fever, twitching.

KIDNEY LINE   SHEN WEN

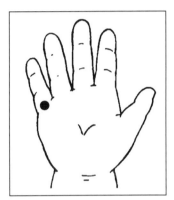

Location: Root of the little finger, palmar transverse crease.

Technique: Press rotate 100–500 times, *or* press 100–300 times.

Action: Expel wind, brighten eyes, disperse lumps and stagnation, clear stagnant heat, lead fire outward.

Indications: Red eyes, thrush, toxic heat syndromes, conjunctivitis, myotic stomatitis, internal heat with external cold.

KIDNEY MERIDIAN   SHEN JING   K

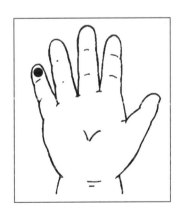

Location: Little fingertip, palmar pad.

Technique: *Tonify:* Press rotate 100–500 times. *Clear:* Push distal to proximal.

Action: *Tonify:* Strengthen kidney and yang. *Clear:* Purge stagnant heat in lower burner.

Indications: Congenital deficiencies, postillness weakness, morning diarrhea, enuresis, cough, asthma, frequent urination, dysuria, convulsions, epilepsy, toothache, five flaccidities, five retardations, paralysis aftermath.

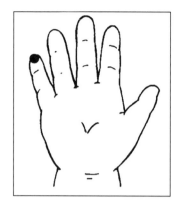

Kidney Summit   Shen ding

Location: Little fingertip.

Technique: Press rotate 100–500 times; *or* fingernail press 5–10 times, then press rotate 50–100 times.

Action: Astringe primary essence, tonify exterior, stop perspiration.

Indications: Spontaneous and/or night sweating, delayed fontanel closure.

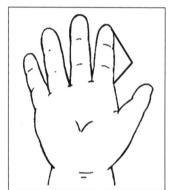

Large Intestine Meridian   Da chang jing   LI

Location: Index finger, medial edge from the tip to the web.

Technique: *Tonify:* Push from distal to proximal 100–500 times. *Clear:* Push from proximal to distal 100–500 times.

Action: *Tonify:* Regulate large intestine function. *Clear:* Disperse large intestine heat, relax bowels.

Indications: Diarrhea, dysentery, constipation, abdominal pain, anal swelling and redness.

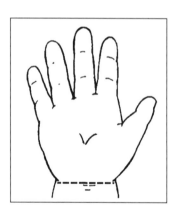

Large Transverse Line   Da heng wen

Location: Palmar wrist crease.

Technique: 1. Press rotate 100–500 times. 2. Push apart 100–300 times. 3. Push converge 100–300 times.

Action: 1. Expel wind, depress perverse qi, balance yin/yang, remove food stagnation. 2. Balance yin/yang, harmonize and regulate zang organs. 3. Resolve phlegm, disperse stagnation.

Indications: 1. Vomiting, alternating chills and fever, asthma with sputum, food stagnation, abdominal distension, diarrhea. 2. Convulsions, epilepsy, coma, twitching, food retention, diarrhea, dysentery. 3. Excess phlegm.

LESSER MARSH   SHAO ZE   SI 1

Location: Little finger, ulnar side, just below the corner of the nail.

Technique: Fingernail press heavily 5–10 times.

Action: Induce perspiration, reduce fever, clear throat, resolve phlegm, stop cough, clear small intestine and heart heat.

Indications: Headache, cough, fever without perspiration, thrush, throat inflammation, swollen tongue.

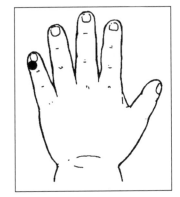

LESSER METAL SOUND   SHAO SHANG   LU 11

Location: Thumb, radial side, just below the corner of the nail.

Technique: Fingernail press heavily 5–10 times.

Action: Expel wind, relieve exterior, clear heat, eliminate vexation, resolve phlegm or dampness.

Indications: Common cold, cough, swelling, throat pain, thrush, dyspnea (phlegm), vexation, restlessness, thirst, chest oppression, vomiting, hiccups, malaria.

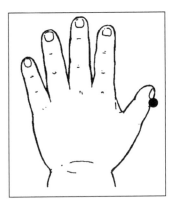

LIVER MERIDIAN   GAN JING   LV

Location: Index finger, palmar pad of the distal phalange.

Technique:* Push proximal to distal 100–500 times, *or* push back and forth 100–300 times.

Action: Clear liver/gallbladder heat, ease mind, relieve convulsions, quell liver, expel wind, reduce fever, relieve depressed liver qi.

Indications: Convulsions, red eyes, anxiety, restlessness, fright, irritability, hot soles or palms, liver wind, sore throat, conjunctivitis, twitching with high fever, thrush, dysuria, deep-colored urine, diarrhea, abdominal distension.

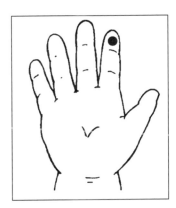

---

* Clinically, it is uncommon to tonify Liver Meridian. If necessary, this can be accomplished by tonifying Kidney Meridian. An exception may be when treating mumps.

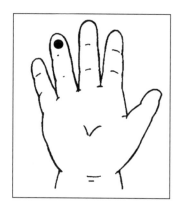

LUNG MERIDIAN   FEI JING   LU

Location: Fourth (ring) finger, pad of the distal phalange.

Technique: *Clear:* Push distal to proximal 100–500 times. *Tonify:* Rotate press 100–500 times.

Action: Facilitate throat, stop cough, smooth qi, resolve phlegm, relax bowels. *Tonify:* Strengthen lungs. *Clear:* Expel excess lung heat.

Indications: Common cold, cough, asthma with sputum, constipation, fever, stuffy chest, dyspnea (phlegm), dry throat.

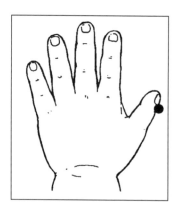

MATERNAL CHEEK   MU SAI

Location: Inferior to the thumbnail, midpoint on the midline.

Technique: Fingernail press 3–5 times.

Action: Stop bleeding and vomiting.

Indications: Bleeding, vomiting.

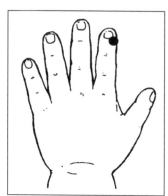

METAL SOUND   SHANG YANG   LI 1

Location: Index finger, radial side, below the corner of the nail.

Technique: Fingernail press heavily 5–10 times.

Action: Expel wind, disperse heat, ventilate and rectify lung qi, resolve phlegm, smooth qi flow.

Indications: Chills and fever, malaria, fever without perspiration, deafness, dry mouth, constipation, oppression, cough, dyspnea.

Nursing the Aged Yang lao SI 6

Location: Dorsal ulnar head, depression on the radial side of the ulnar styloid process.

Technique: Fingernail press 3–5 times, then grasp 10–15 times.

Action: Tonify spleen, calm fright, reduce fever.

Indications: Dyspepsia, palpitation (fright), hectic fever.

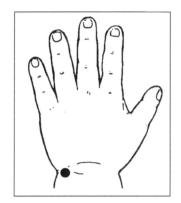

Old Dragon Lao long

Location: Inferior to the middle fingernail, midpoint on the midline.

Technique: Fingernail press 3–10 times.

Action: Resuscitate from unconsciousness, stop convulsions, reduce fever and pathological fire, open orifices, recuperate yang.

Indications: Acute febrile convulsions, fever, irritability, fright, restlessness, afternoon fever, dull mind, wailing, coma.

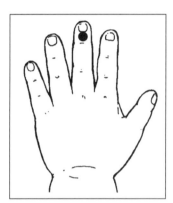

One Nestful Wind Yi wo feng

Location: Dorsal wrist, midpoint on the transverse crease.

Technique: Press rotate 100–300 times, *or* fingernail press 10–20 times, *or* push apart 50–100 times (push apart provides less intense stimulation than the fingernail press).

Action: Warm middle burner, increase qi circulation, relieve abdominal pain, relieve joint pain, expel wind cold, warm and connect interior with exterior, calm fright, ease mind, relieve pain, relieve external symptoms.

Indications: Abdominal pain, borborygmus, common cold, swelling and painful joints, convulsions, arthralgia.

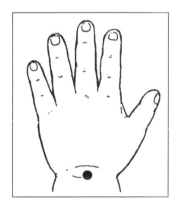

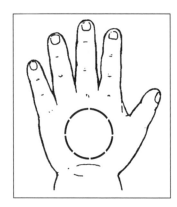

OUTER EIGHT SYMBOLS   WAI BA GUA

Location: Dorsal hand, circle around External Palace of Labor (opposite Inner Eight Symbols).

Technique: Rotate push 300–500 times, moving around the child's left hand clockwise and the child's right hand counterclockwise.

Action: Drive qi, harmonize blood, remove and disperse stagnation.

Indications: Chest oppression, abdominal distension, constipation, zang-fu disharmony, qi or blood stagnation.

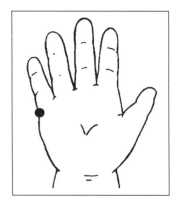

PALMAR SMALL TRANSVERSE LINE   ZHENG XIAO HENG WEN

Location: Base of the little finger, palmar side, ulnar edge of the transverse line.

Technique: Press rotate 100–300 times, *or* push back and forth 100–300 times.

Action: Clear heat, disperse stagnation, ventilate lungs, resolve cough and phlegm.

Indications: Dyspnea (phlegm), cough, fever, thrush.

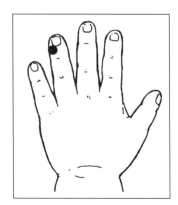

PASSAGE HUB   GUAN CHONG   TW 1

Location: Fourth finger, ulnar side, below the corner of the nail.

Technique: Fingernail press heavily 5–10 times.

Action: Clear head and eyes, facilitate triple burner, relieve chest and diaphragm, ease mind.

Indications: Headache, dullness, poor vision, dry mouth, sore throat, choking, anorexia.

SMALL CELESTIAL CENTER   XIAO TIAN XIN

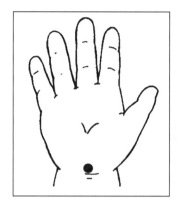

Location: Base of the palm at the junction of the major and minor thenars, just above the wrist transverse line.

Technique: Press rotate 100–300 times, *or* pound 30–100 times, *or* fingernail press 3–5 times.

Action: Clear orifices, eliminate stagnation, stop convulsions, ease mind, brighten eyes, clear pathogenic heat, promote urination, calm fright, disperse stagnation.

Indications: Convulsions, epilepsy, blurred vision, eye redness, eye pain and swelling, excess tears, unclosed fontanel, high fever, coma, vexation, restlessness, night crying, insomnia, anuria, incomplete measles or pox.

SMALL INTESTINE MERIDIAN   XIAO CHANG JING   SI

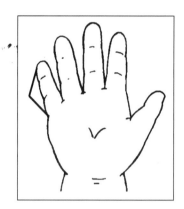

Location: Little finger, ulnar edge from the tip to the root.

Technique:* *Clear:* Push proximal to distal 100–500 times.

Action: Clear heat, promote urination, clear heart pathogenic heat invading small intestine.

Indications: Diarrhea, scant urine, anuria, high fever, afternoon fever, enuresis, dark urine, thrush.

SMALL TRANSVERSE LINES   SUI HENG WEN

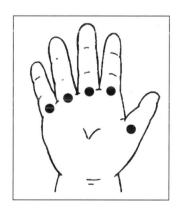

Location: All five fingers at the palmar transverse lines where the fingers join the palm.

Technique: Fingernail press 2–5 times, *or* push back and forth 50–100 times, *or* press rotate 100–300 times.

Action: Clear heat, eliminate vexation, disperse stagnation, resolve phlegm.

Indications: Fever, fretfulness, thrush, cough, dyspnea.

---

* Clinically, Small Intestine Meridian is usually not tonified.

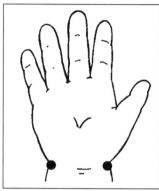

SNAIL SHELL   LUO SI

Location: Bilateral distal ends of the ulnar and radial bones at the extreme medial and lateral points.

Technique: Press rotate (two fingers) 100–500 times.

Action: Relieve cough, depress adverse rising qi.

Indications: Cough, asthma, EPI.

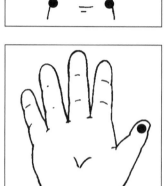

SPLEEN MERIDIAN   PI JING   SP

Location: Thumb at the distal phalange.

Technique: *Tonify:* Press rotate 300–500 times. *Clear:* Push proximal to distal 300–500 times.

Action: *Tonify:* Strengthen stomach and spleen, tonify blood, resolve phlegm. *Clear:* Remove food stagnation, promote digestion, eliminate dampness.

Indications: Spleen and stomach deficiency, anorexia, emaciation, listlessness, diarrhea, indigestion, constipation, poor appetite, dysentery, convulsions, damp phlegm, jaundice, abdominal distension, spontaneous sweating, night sweats, muscle atrophy, incomplete measles or pox.

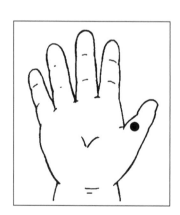

STOMACH MERIDIAN   WEI JING   ST

Location: Thumb, palmar side, second segment.

Technique: *Tonify:* Press rotate 300–500 times. *Clear:* Push proximal to distal 300–500 times.

Action: Stop vomiting, depress adverse rising qi, promote digestion, clear heat.

Indications: Vomiting, hiccups, thirst, poor appetite, pathological stomach fire, abdominal distension, anorexia, diarrhea.

SWEET LOAD   GAN ZAI

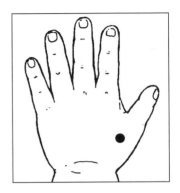

Location: Dorsal hand, proximal to Union Valley, at the intersection of the first and second metacarpals.

Technique: Fingernail press 5–10 times, then press rotate 50–100 times.

Action: Recuperate yang, resuscitate from unconsciousness.

Indications: Convulsions, swooning, sudden faint, cold extremities.

SYMMETRIC UPRIGHT   DUAN ZHENG

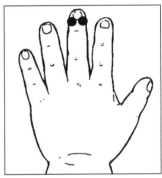

Location: Middle finger, bilateral points at the corners of the nail.

Technique: Fingernail press (bilateral) 5–10 times, *or* press rotate 10–20 times.

Action: Clear heart and liver fire, calm fright, ease mind, depress adverse rising qi, tonify spleen, harmonize stomach. *Radial:* Tonify ascending qi. *Ulnar:* Tonify descending qi.

Indications: Convulsions. *Radial:* Diarrhea, dysentery. *Ulnar:* Vomiting, epistaxis.

TEN KINGS   SHI WANG   X 24

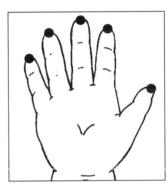

Location: Tips of all five fingers.

Technique: Fingernail press 3–5 times.

Action: Resuscitate from unconsciousness, reduce fever, calm fright, ease mind, clear fire, relieve spasms, eliminate vexation.

Indications: Acute convulsions, dull mind, night crying, spasms, high fever, fretfulness, restlessness.

THREE DIGITAL PASSES   ZHI SAN GUAN

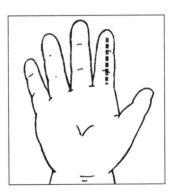

Location: Index finger, palmar side, three segments: Wind (proximal), Qi (middle), Vital (distal).

Technique:* Push distal to proximal 100–200 times.

Action: Harmonize blood, dredge passes, quench liver/gallbladder fire, clear large intestine heat.

Indications: Fever, cold aversion, diarrhea, dysentery, convulsions.

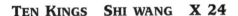

* Clinically, Three Digital Passes is used more often for assessment than treatment; see chapter 5.

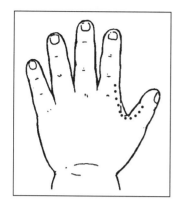

TIGER'S MOUTH   HU KOU

Location: The web between the thumb and index finger, from the index knuckle to the thumb's second joint.

 This point is used as a landmark in technique descriptions (for example, "Celestial Gate to Tiger's Mouth").

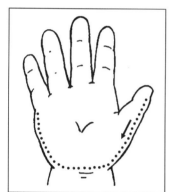

TRANSPORT EARTH TO WATER   YUN TU RU SHUI

Location: From the radial tip of the thumb along the edge of the palm in a curve to the little finger.

Technique: Push with thumb 100–300 times.

Action: Clear stomach/spleen damp heat, replenish insufficient water, supplement kidney water.

Indications: Diarrhea, abdominal distension, borborygmus, indigestion, vomiting, dysentery.

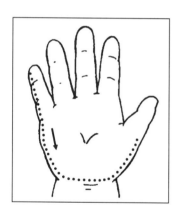

TRANSPORT WATER TO EARTH   YUN SHUI RU TU

Location: From the little finger root along the edge of the palm to the medial thumb.

Technique: Push with thumb 100–300 times.

Action: Moisten dryness, promote bowel movement, promote urination, tonify spleen, promote digestion, remove stagnation.

Indications: Dysuria, yellow urine, constipation, weak constitution, abdominal distension, malnutrition, anorexia, diarrhea, dysentery, food retention.

TWO HORSES   ER MA

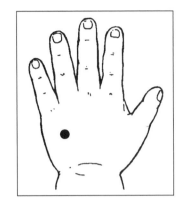

Location: Dorsal hand on the ulnar side of the center (External Palace of Labor), between the fourth and fifth fingers.

Technique: Press rotate 100–300 times, *or* fingernail press 5–10 times.

Action: Tonify or reinforce kidney yin, tonify kidney yang, retrieve yang, lead fire to original place, drive qi, disperse stagnation.

Indications: Dysuria, indigestion, abdominal pain, weak constitution, prolapsed rectum, enuresis, cough, asthma, dark urine, toothache, phlegm dampness, teeth grinding, coma, lumbago, tinnitus, leg flaccidity, neck swelling or pain.

TWO LEAF DOORS   ER SHAN MEN

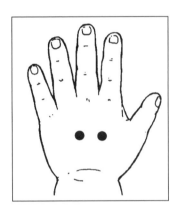

Location: Dorsal hand, the two depressions on either side of the center (External Palace of Labor).

Technique: Press both points 3–5 times, *or* press rotate 300–500 times.

Action: Promote diaphoresis, relieve exterior, promote smooth circulation of qi and blood to relax muscles and tendons, expel wind, clear collaterals, relieve dyspnea.

Indications: Febrile symptoms due to pathogenic wind or cold, anhidrosis, asthma with sputum, stuffy chest, convulsions, febrile with no sweating, common cold, dyspnea (phlegm), cough, incomplete measles or pox.

UNION VALLEY   HE GU   LI 4

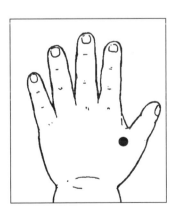

Location: Dorsal hand, between the first and second metacarpals on the radial aspect, at the end of the crease in the web between the thumb and index finger.

Technique: Press rotate 100–200 times; *or* fingernail press 3–5 times, then press rotate 50–100 times.

Action: Induce perspiration, relieve exterior, disperse stagnation, clear heat, relieve pain.

Indications: Headache, stiff neck, fever without perspiration, epistaxis, sore throat, toothache, trismus, constipation, vomiting, adverse rising of qi.

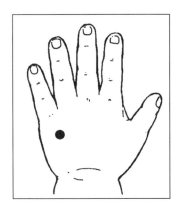

VIM TRANQUILLITY   JING NING

Location: Dorsal hand, at the depression behind the fourth and fifth metacarpals, and on the ulnar side of External Palace of Labor.

Technique: Press 3–5 times, then rub; *or* fingernail press 3–5 times, then press rotate 100–300 times.

Action: Promote digestion, remove food stagnation, relieve chest, facilitate diaphragm, drive qi.

Indications: Asthma with sputum, retching, abdominal lumps, chest or abdominal fullness, stagnant accumulation, dyspnea (phlegm), wheezing.

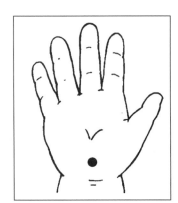

WATER (INNER EIGHT SYMBOLS)   KAN GONG

Location: Palm, at the six o'clock point in Inner Eight Symbols (see page 62).

Technique: Fingernail press 10–20 times, *or* push 100–200 times.

Action: Promote diaphoresis, relieve exterior.

Indications: External pathogenic influences, lung distress.

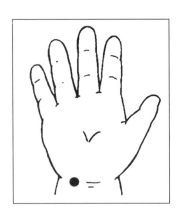

WHITE TENDON   BAI JIN

Location: Palmar transverse wrist crease, midway between Chief Tendon (midpoint) and Yin Pool (lesser thenar eminence).

Technique: Fingernail press 3–5 times, *or* press rotate 50–100 times.

Action: Smooth qi flow, resolve phlegm, relieve chest, facilitate diaphragm.

Indications: Chest oppression, dyspnea (phlegm).

WOOD GATE   BAN MEN

Location: At the center of the greater thenar eminence (0.5 cun inferior to the second phalange joint of the thumb).

Technique: *Tonify:* Press rotate 100–300 times. *Clear:* Push 100–200 times.

Action: Relieve convulsions, remove food stagnation, promote digestion, drain excess heat of stomach and spleen, tonify spleen, harmonize stomach, cool diaphragm.

Indications: Acute or chronic convulsions, opisthotonos, indigestion, vomiting, diarrhea, shortness of breath.

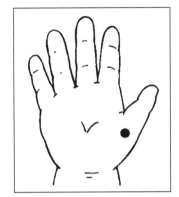

YANG MARSH   YANG XI   LI 5

Location: Radial end of the dorsal transverse wrist crease.

Technique: Fingernail press 5–10 times, then press rotate 50–100 times.

Action: Control malaria, stop diarrhea.

Indications: Malaria, diarrhea.

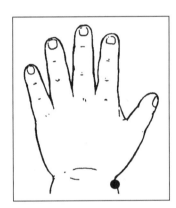

YIN POOL   YIN QI

Location: Lesser thenar eminence (the corner at the lowest edge of the palm, ulnar side).

This point is used as a landmark in technique descriptions (for example, swift-shifting press).

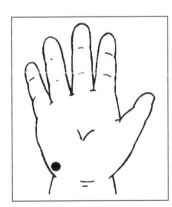

Arm Region

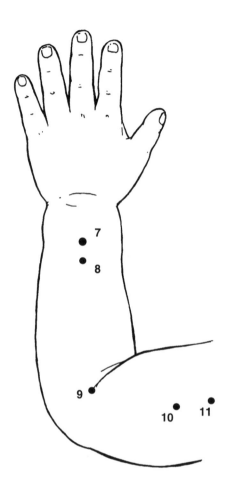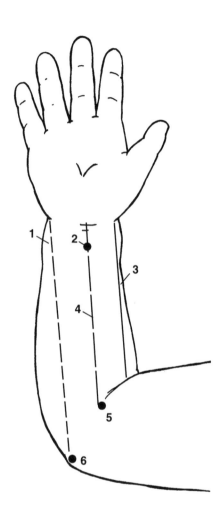

ARM-POINT NAMES

8	Arm Yang Pool	9	Pool at the Bend	10	Upper Arm
2	Inner Pass	11	Shoulder Bone	5	Vast Pool
6	Lesser Sea	1	Six Hollow Bowels	4	Water of Galaxy
7	Outer Pass	3	Three Passes		

Arm Yang Pool   Bo yang qi

Location: 3 cun superior to the center of the dorsal transverse wrist crease (One Nestful Wind).

Technique: Press rotate 300–500 times; *or* fingernail press 5–7 times, then press rotate 10–30 times.

Action: Depress adverse rising qi, lead fire downward, disperse heat.

Indications: Dizziness, headache, convulsions, epilepsy, constipation, dysuria, dark urine, dry stool, diarrhea, enuresis.

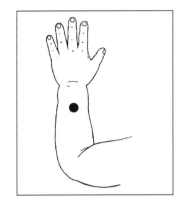

Inner Pass   Nei guan   P 6

Location: 2 cun superior to the transverse crease of the wrist on the medial aspect of the forearm, between the two tendons.

Technique: Fingernail press 10–20 times, *or* press rotate 100–200 times.

Action: Promote diaphoresis, relieve exterior.

Indications: External pathogenic influences.

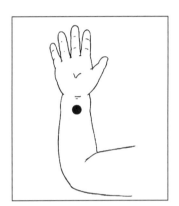

Lesser Sea   Shao hai   H 3

Location: Between the ulnar end of the elbow transverse line and the medial humeral epicondyle.

Technique: Press rotate 30–50 times; *or* fingernail press 3–5 times, then press rotate 30–35 times; *or* grasp and rock 30–50 times.

Action: Smooth qi flow, activate blood.

Indications: Chest and abdominal stuffiness or fullness, convulsions.

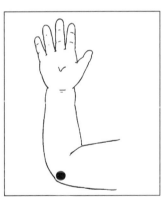

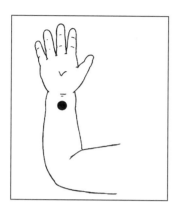

OUTER PASS   WAI GUAN   TW 5

Location: 2 cun superior to the dorsal wrist transverse crease, between the radius and the ulna.

Technique: Press rotate 100–300 times, *or* fingernail press 3–7 times, then press rotate 50–100 times.

Action: Expel wind, disperse cold, relieve pain.

Indications: Diarrhea, back pain, lumbago, common cold, cold aversion.

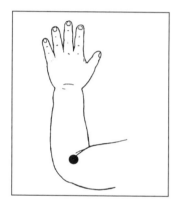

POOL AT THE BEND   QU QI   LI 11

Location: With the elbow flexed, the lateral end of the elbow transverse crease.

Technique: Fingernail press 5–7 times, then press rotate 30–50 times.

Action: Eliminate stagnation, induce perspiration, relieve exterior, clear heat, relieve pain.

Indications: Upper extremities numb or disabled, finger pain with movement, common cold, fever, belching, vomiting, cough, dyspnea.

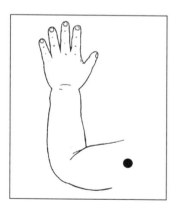

SHOULDER BONE   JIAN YU   LI 15

Location: The depression that appears at the anterior border of the acromioclavicular joint when the arm is raised laterally and abducted.

Technique: Press rotate 100–300 times.

Action: Relax tendons, open channels and collaterals.

Indications: Convulsions, stiffness and atrophy of upper limbs.

SIX HOLLOW BOWELS LIU FU

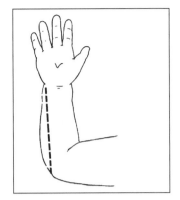

Location: Lower edge of the ulnar bone from the elbow to the wrist crease.

Technique: Push proximal to distal 100–500 times.

Action: Clear heat, cool blood, detoxify, resolve swelling, relieve pain.

Indications: High fever, irritability, dry stools, thirst, desire for cold drinks, febrile syndromes, convulsions, thrush, swollen tongue, gum ulcers, throat pain, swelling, mumps, sores, depressed heat, stagnant accumulation in bowels, dysentery, constipation.

THREE PASSES SAN GUAN

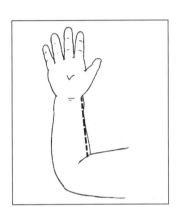

Location: Radial border of the forearm, from the wrist crease to the elbow joint.

Technique: Push distal to proximal 100–500 times (increase this number for cold patterns).

Action: Reinforce qi, tonify yang, disperse pathogenic cold, relieve exterior syndromes, tonify deficiency, promote flow of qi, activate blood, clear collaterals, cultivate and supplement essence.

Indications:* Abdominal pain, diarrhea, postillness weakness, cold aversion, weak limbs, anorexia, jaundice, anemia, incomplete measles or pox, polio, ulcer, furuncle, spontaneous perspiration, deficient qi and blood, weak constitution, yang deficiency.

UPPER ARM BI NAO LI 14

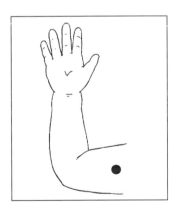

Location: Upper arm at the lateral midline, just superior to the insertion of the deltoid muscle.

Technique: Press rotate 100–300 times.

Action: Relax and relieve eye muscle tension.

Indications: Eye problems, strabismus, crossed eyes.

---

* Contraindications: Excess heat syndromes.

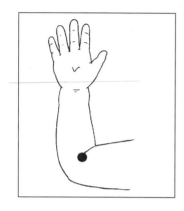

Vast Pool   Hong qi

Location: Elbow transverse crease, ulnar side of the biceps brachii tendon.

Technique: Press rotate 50–100 times; *or* grasp 3–5 times; *or* fingernail press 3–5 times, then press rotate 10–20 times.

Action: Ease mind, calm fright, clear pericardium heat.

Indications: Twitching of upper extremities, convulsions.

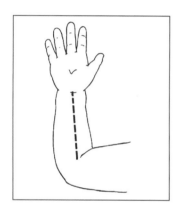

Water of Galaxy   Tian he shui

Location: Forearm, medial aspect, at the midline, from the wrist crease to the elbow crease.

Technique: Push distal to proximal 100–500 times.

Action: Clear pathogenic heat and fire, relieve exterior, clear heart heat, eliminate vexation and fretfulness, calm fright, resolve excess and deficiency heat syndromes.

Indications: Deficient yin heat, febrile syndrome, common-cold fever, tidal fever, excess internal heat, irritability, restlessness, thirst, stiff tongue, convulsions, fright crying, fretfulness, abdominal distension, stomach/spleen heat, myotic stomatitis, thrush, swollen gums, ulcer, cough, dyspnea (phlegm), dry stool, dark urine, excess and heat syndromes.

Anterior Torso Region

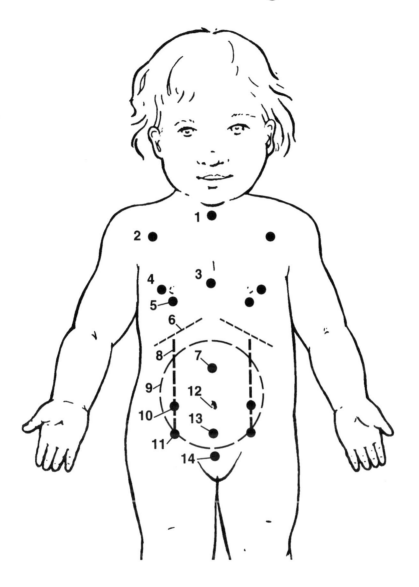

ANTERIOR TORSO-POINT NAMES

9	Abdomen	5	Breast Root	14	Curved Bone
7	Abdominal Center	1	Celestial Chimney	13	Elixir Field
11	Abdominal Corner	10	Celestial Pivot	4	Outside Nipple
6	Abdominal Yin Yang	2	Central Treasury	12	Spirit Gate
8	Below Ribs	3	Chest Center		

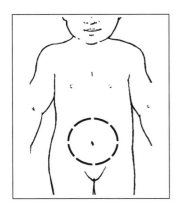

ABDOMEN FU

Location: Epigastric region

Technique: Rotate push 36 rotations clockwise then 36 counterclockwise. Repeat for 5–7 minutes, *or* push apart from midline to side 50–100 times.

Action: Promote digestion, warm yang, tonify stomach and spleen, regulate gastrointestinal functions, relieve dyspepsia, disperse stagnant qi, relieve abdominal pain or distension.

Indications: Abdominal pain, indigestion, vomiting, diarrhea, constipation, abdominal distension or pain, borborygmus, food retention, malnutrition.

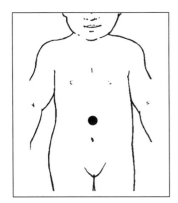

ABDOMINAL CENTER ZHONG WAN CV 12

Location: At the abdominal midline, halfway between the navel and the xiphoid process.

Technique: Press rotate 100–200 times, *or* push from Celestial Chimney to Abdominal Center.

Action: Tonify stomach/spleen, promote digestion.

Indications: Abdominal distension, indigestion, diarrhea, appetite loss, belching, dyspnea, dyspepsia, vomiting, stomachache.

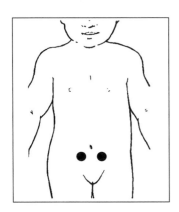

ABDOMINAL CORNER DU JIAO

Location: 2 cun inferior and lateral to the navel.

Technique: Grasp 3–5 times.

Action: Relieve abdominal pain due to pathogenic cold or irregular diet, disperse cold, clear heat, disperse stagnation, stop diarrhea, relax bowels.

Indications: Abdominal pain (especially pathogenic cold), diarrhea, constipation, dysentery.

ABDOMINAL YIN YANG   FU YIN YANG

Location: Upper abdominal quadrants.

Technique: Rotate push 100–200 times, *or* push apart 50–300 times.

Action: Tonify stomach/spleen, promote digestion, promote qi flow, relieve pain, stop vomiting, stop diarrhea.

Indications: Abdominal pain or distension, indigestion, vomiting, nausea, dyspepsia, diarrhea.

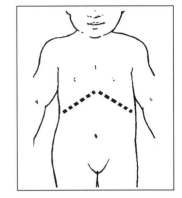

BELOW RIBS   XIE LEI

Location: Inferior to the costal ridge on the vertical nipple line, from the costal ridge to Abdominal Corner.

Technique:* Push superior to inferior 100–300 times.

Action: Regulate qi flow, resolve phlegm, regulate large intestine, remove food stagnation, eliminate distension, promote digestion.

Indications: Indigestion, stuffy chest, abdominal distension (phlegm), stagnant food retention, abdominal pain, constipation, borborygmus.

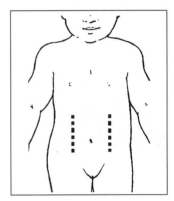

BREAST ROOT   RU GEN   ST 18

Location: Inferior to the nipples by one rib space (fifth intercostal space).

Technique: Press rotate 50–100 times.

Action: Regulate lung qi, resolve cough and phlegm.

Indications: Asthma, cough, stuffy chest.

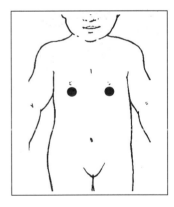

---

* Shifting your emphasis medially, closer to the midline, is more useful for diarrhea.

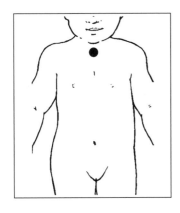

CELESTIAL CHIMNEY TIAN TU CV 22

Location: Center of the suprasternal fossa, superior to the suprasternal notch.

Technique: Press rotate 30–50 times, *or* pinch squeeze 3–5 times, *or* fingernail press 3–5 times.

Action: Clear phlegm obstruction, clear heat, facilitate throat, depress adverse rising qi, relieve dyspnea, stop vomiting.

Indications: Dyspnea, sore throat, hoarseness, insufficient phlegm discharge, cough, sudden aphonia, vomiting.

First aid: Forceful pressure will induce vomiting.

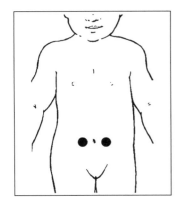

CELESTIAL PIVOT TIAN SHU ST 25

Location: 2 cun lateral to the navel.

Technique: * Press rotate 50–100 times, *or* grasp 3–5 times, *or* push (downward) from Celestial Pivot 30–50 times (for moving stagnant food).

Action: Regulate large intestine, regulate qi circulation, remove food stagnation, promote fluid transportation, eliminate distension, promote digestion.

Indications: Abdominal pain, diarrhea, constipation, abdominal distension, indigestion by food stagnation, borborygmus, dysentery, edema.

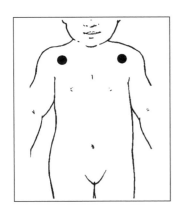

CENTRAL TREASURY ZHONG FU LU 1

Location: Lateral and superior to the sternum at the lateral side of the first intercostal space.

Technique: Press rotate 100–300 times, *or* pinch squeeze until red.

Action: Tonify lung, clear congestion, disperse accumulation.

Indications: Lung distress, pneumonia.

---

* See also Below Ribs.

CHEST CENTER DAN ZHONG CV 17

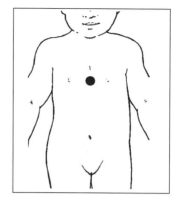

Location: At the chest midline between the nipples (level with the fourth intercostal space).

Technique: Press rotate 30–60 times, *or* pinch squeeze 30–60 times, *or* push apart 50–100 times, *or* push (downward) 50–100 times.

Action: Regulate lung qi, stop cough, relieve chest, smooth qi flow, relieve dyspnea.

Indications: Chest congestion, asthma, cough, vomiting, nausea, dyspnea (phlegm), wheeze, diaphragm distension, hiccups, phlegm, bronchitis.

CURVED BONE QU GU CV 2

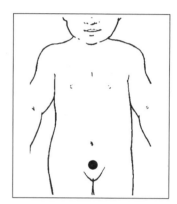

Location: Midpoint of the pubic bone at its upper border.

Technique: Press rotate 200–500 times.

Action: Tonify kidney, tonify lower burner.

Indications: Enuresis.

ELIXIR FIELD DAN TIAN

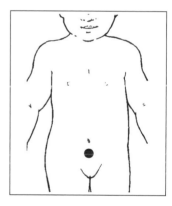

Location: 3 cun inferior to the navel on the midline.

Technique: Press rotate 100–300 times, *or* rotate push 30–50 times.

Action: Tonify kidney.

Indications: Diarrhea, abdominal pain, enuresis, prolapsed rectum, hernia, anuria, congenital qi deficiency.

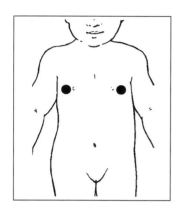

OUTSIDE NIPPLE   RU PANG

Location: Lateral to each nipple.

Technique: Press rotate 30–50 times.

Action: Relax chest, facilitate qi flow.

Indications: Cough, dyspnea (phlegm), chest oppression or pain, dysphagia.

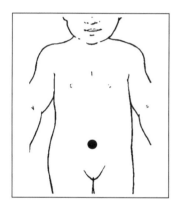

SPIRIT GATE   SHEN QUE   CV 8

Location: Navel.

Technique: Press rotate 100–500 times, *or* rotate push 100–300 times.

Action: Warm yang, tonify deficiency, tonify spleen to relieve diarrhea, regulate gastrointestinal function, relieve dyspepsia, disperse stagnant qi, promote digestion, relieve abdominal pain.

Indications: Dyspepsia, borborygmus, indigestion, food retention, malnutrition. *Tonify:* Spleen deficiency, diarrhea, indigestion, abdominal distension. *Clear:* Constipation, indigestion, abdominal distension and pain.

Posterior Torso Region

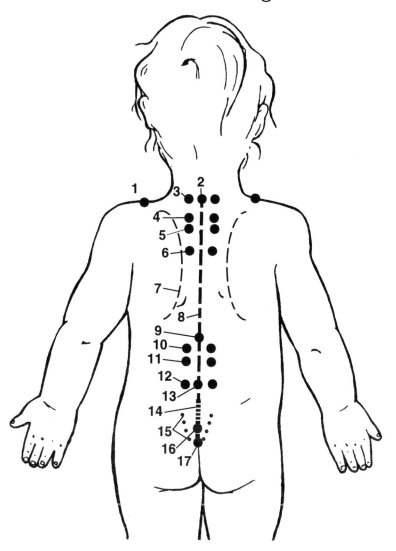

POSTERIOR TORSO-POINT NAMES

14	Bone of Seven Segments	12	Kidney Back Point	8	Spinal Column
3	Calm Breath	13	Life Gate	10	Spleen Back Point
9	Central Pivot	16	Lumbar Back Point	11	Stomach Back Point
15	Eight Sacral Holes	5	Lung Back Point	17	Tortoise Tail
2	Great Hammer	7	Scapula	4	Wind Gate
6	Heart Back Point	1	Shoulder Well		

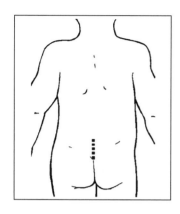

BONE OF SEVEN SEGMENTS   QI JIE GU

Location: Sacral midline, from L-2 (Life Gate) to the coccyx (Tortoise Tail).

Technique: Push 100–300 times, *or* rotate push 100–200 times, *or* chafe until warm.

Action: Relax bowels, stop diarrhea, relieve constipation. *Push (downward):* Relieve constipation. *Push (upward):* Stop diarrhea.

Indications: Diarrhea, constipation, dysentery, prolapsed rectum. *Push (downward):* Constipation. *Push (upward):* Diarrhea.

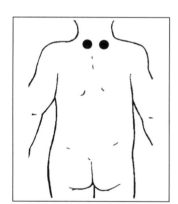

CALM BREATH   DING CHUAN   X 14

Location: Upper back, 0.5 cun lateral to Great Hammer.

Technique: Press rotate 100–300 times.

Action: Relieve cough, disperse stagnant lung qi, facilitate lung.

Indications: Asthma, cough, rubella.

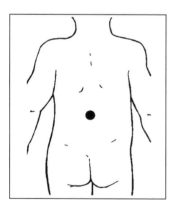

CENTRAL PIVOT   ZHONG SHU   GV 7

Location: Midline of the back, between T-10 and T-11.

Technique: Press rotate 50–100 times.

Action: Tonify kidney, consolidate waist.

Indications: Lumbago, stiff spine, difficulty flexing or extending the back.

EIGHT SACRAL HOLES   BA LIAO   BL 31~34

Location: At the sacrum, the four foramen (holes) on each side of the midline.

Technique: Chafe until warm.

Action: Tonify, warm, and consolidate lower burner.

Indications: Enuresis.

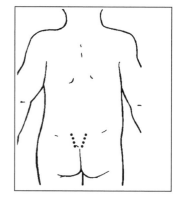

GREAT HAMMER   DA ZHUI   GV 14

Location: Upper back midline between C-7 and T-1.

Technique: Press rotate 50–100 times.

Action: Induce perspiration, relieve exterior, relieve dyspnea, stop vomiting, clear heat, expel wind, relax spasms, remove exogenous attack, clear heart and lung heat.

Indications: Exogenous fever, stiff neck, dyspnea, vomiting, diarrhea, convulsions, opisthotonos, common cold, shoulder pain.

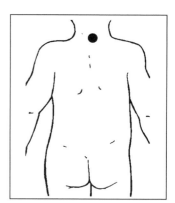

HEART BACK POINT   XIN SHU   BL 15

Location: 1.5 cun lateral to the midline of the spine, at the level of the T-5 vertebra.

Technique: Press rotate 50–100 times.

Action: Tonify heart, clear excess heat, calm spirit.

Indications: Agitation, convulsions, excess-heat syndromes.

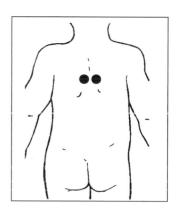

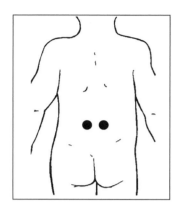

KIDNEY BACK POINT   SHEN SHU   BL 23

Location: Lower back, at the level of L-2, 1.5 cun lateral to the spine bilaterally.

Technique: Press rotate 100–300 times.

Action: Tonify kidney, warm yang, supplement and tonify essence.

Indications: Kidney deficiency, diarrhea, enuresis, limb weakness.

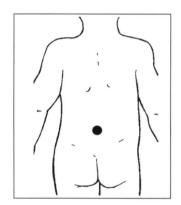

LIFE GATE   MING MEN   GV 4

Location: At the midline of the lower back, inferior to the L-2 spinous process.

Technique: Press rotate 100–300 times, *or* chafe until warm.

Action: Tonify kidney, warm yang, supplement and tonify essence.

Indications: Enuresis, kidney deficiency or weakness.

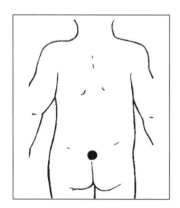

LUMBAR BACK POINT   YAO SHU   GV 2

Location: Lower back, inferior to S-4, in the hiatus sacralalis.

Technique: Press rotate 100–300 times, *or* chafe until warm.

Action: Relax tendons, activate blood, tonify kidney.

Indications: Lumbago, diarrhea, limb flaccidity.

LUNG BACK POINT   FEI SHU   BL 13

Location: Upper back, 1.5 cun lateral to T-3 bilaterally.

Technique: Press rotate 100–200 times, *or* push (downward) along scapula border 100–300 times, *or* push apart 50–100 times.

Action: Clear lung heat, tonify deficiency, stop cough, relieve dyspnea, regulate lung qi.

Indications: Lung heat, dyspnea, accumulated depressed fire in chest, common cold, cough, lung deficiency due to protracted cough.

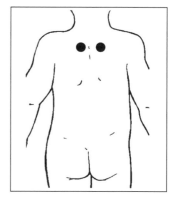

SCAPULA   JIAN JIE GU

Location: Both scapulae, including the area between them.

Technique: Push apart, moving from superior to inferior along the scapula border, and reverse; repeat 100–300 times.

Action: Disperse excess lung qi, resolve cough, relieve asthma.

Indications: Lung qi dysfunction, cough, asthma.

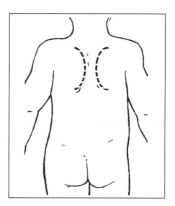

SHOULDER WELL   JIAN JING   GB 21

Location: Upper back, at the midpoint between Great Hammer (C-7) and the acromial process on the highest point of the shoulder.

Technique: Grasp 5–10 times, *or* press 5–10 times.

Action: Relax tendons and ligaments, improve qi and blood circulation, lower rebellious qi.

Indications: Neck rigidity, adverse rising of qi.

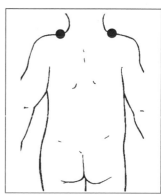

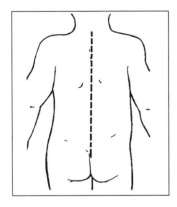

SPINAL COLUMN JI ZHU

Location: Midline of the back, from Great Hammer to Tortoise Tail (the coccyx).

Technique: Push superior to inferior 300–500 times, *or* spinal pinch pull inferior to superior 3–5 times.

Action: Reduce fever, eliminate distension, tonify stomach/spleen, regulate yin/yang, qi, and blood, harmonize zang-fu, promote smooth meridian function. *Push (downward):* Clear excess. *Spinal pinch pull (upward):* Tonify deficiency.

Indications: Fever, malnutrition, stomach/spleen deficiency, convulsions, night crying, diarrhea, vomiting, abdominal pain, constipation. *Push (downward):* Fever, convulsions. *Spinal pinch pull (upward):* Malnutrition, deficiency diarrhea.

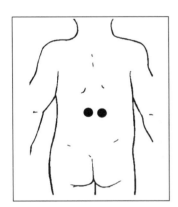

SPLEEN BACK POINT PI SHU BL 20

Location: Middle back, 1.5 cun lateral to the spine at the level of T-11 bilaterally.

Technique: Press rotate 50–100 times.

Action: Tonify stomach/spleen, promote digestion, eliminate dampness, promote food assimilation.

Indications: Vomiting, malnutrition, convulsions, weak limbs, diarrhea, spleen deficiency.

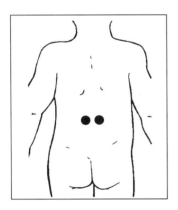

STOMACH BACK POINT WEI SHU BL 21

Location: 1.5 cun lateral to the midline of the spine, at the level of the lower border of the T-12 vertebra.

Technique: Press rotate 50–100 times.

Action: Tonify stomach/spleen, promote digestion, eliminate dampness, clear stomach heat.

Indications: Digestive distress, vomiting.

TORTOISE TAIL GUI WEI GV 1

Location: Inferior to the coccyx tip.

Technique: Press rotate 300–500 times; *or* fingernail press 3–5 times, then press rotate 30–50 times.

Action: Stop diarrhea, relax bowels, calm fright, warm yang.

Indications: Convulsions, constipation, diarrhea, abdominal pain, dysentery, prolapsed rectum.

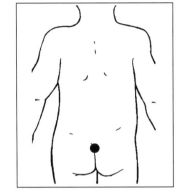

WIND GATE FENG MEN BL 12

Location: Upper back, 1.5 cun lateral to the spine at the level of T-2 bilaterally.

Technique: Press rotate 50–100 times.

Action: Expel wind, disperse cold, clear heat, stop cough, clear meridians, activate collaterals.

Indications: Common cold, cough, dyspnea, fever, headache, stiff neck, back pain, lumbago, asthma.

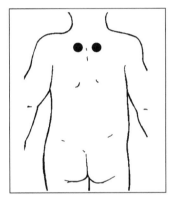

Leg Region

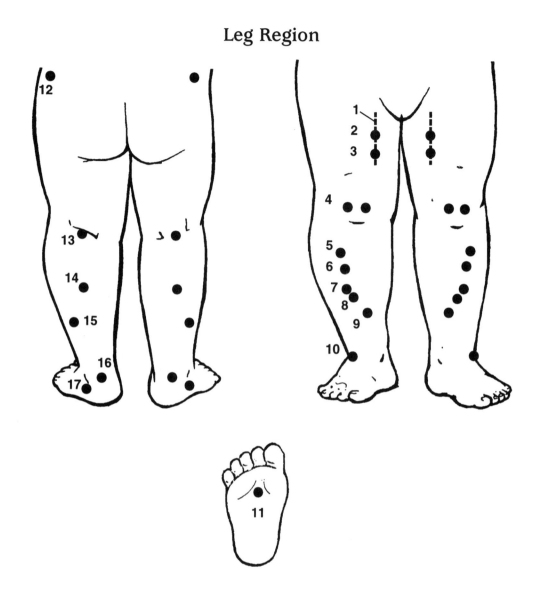

LEG-POINT NAMES					
13	Bend Middle	12	Jumping Round	17	Subservient Visitor
7	Bountiful Bulge	16	Kun Lun Mountains	15	Suspended Bell
11	Bubbling Spring	6	Leg Three Miles	9	Three Yin Meeting
8	Front Mountain Support	14	Mountain Support	1	Winnower Gate
4	Ghost Eye	10	Ravine Divide	5	Yang Mound Spring
2	Hundreds Worms Nest	3	Sea of Blood		

BEND MIDDLE   WEI ZHONG   BL 40

Location: Behind the knee, at the midpoint of the transverse crease.

Technique: Fingernail press heavily 5–10 times.

Action: Dredge or open cold blockage, activate collaterals, expel wind, clear meridians.

Indications: Convulsions, paralysis, blockage syndrome, spasms, weakness or atrophy of lower limbs.

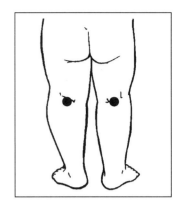

BOUNTIFUL BULGE   FENG LONG   ST 40

Location: Lateral aspect of the lower leg, halfway between the knee and the ankle.

Technique: Press rotate 100–300 times.

Action: Relieve chest, facilitate diaphragm.

Indications: Cough, asthma.

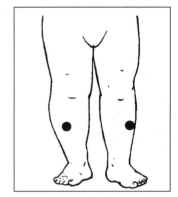

BUBBLING SPRING   YONG QUAN   K 1

Location: Sole of the foot, just below the ball along the longitudinal midline (approximately one-third of the distance from the toes to the heel).

Technique: Press rotate 50–100 times, *or* fingernail press 5–10 times, *or* push with both thumbs from Bubbling Spring to the middle toe 50–100 times.

Action: Clear kidney fire, eliminate fretfulness, lead heat downward, reduce deficient yin fever. *Right foot:* Stop vomiting. *Left foot:* Stop diarrhea.

Indications: Headache, throat inflammation, convulsions, vomiting, diarrhea, dysuria, fever, hot palms or soles, difficult urination, irritability.

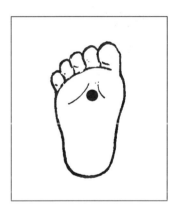

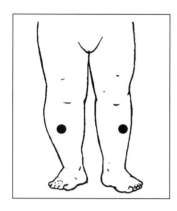

FRONT MOUNTAIN SUPPORT   QIAN CHENG SHAN

Location: Anterior lower leg, approximately halfway between the patella and the ankle on the lateral aspect of the tibia (opposite Mountain Support).

Technique: Fingernail press 10–20 times.

Action: Relax spasms, expel wind.

Indications: Convulsions, opisthotonos (use after Vim Tranquillity and Imposing Agility).

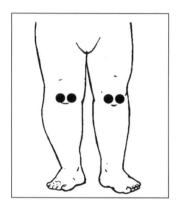

GHOST EYE   GUI YAN

Location: The depression on both sides of the knee, just below the patella.

Technique: Grasp 10–20 times, then press rotate 20–40 times.

Action: Calm fright, relieve spasms, ease mind.

Indications: Convulsions, twitching, weakness, atrophy of lower limbs, spasms.

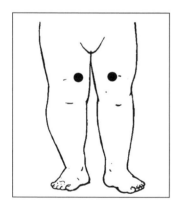

HUNDREDS WORMS NEST   BAI CHONG WO   X 35

Location: 1 cun superior to Sea of Blood, at the medial edge of the femur.

Technique: Grasp 20–40 times.

Action: Calm fright, ease mind, relieve spasms, open orifices, dredge passes.

Indications: Convulsions, coma.

JUMPING ROUND   HUAN TIAO   GB 30

Location: Lateral aspect of the hip, approximately one-third of the distance from the greater trochanter to the sacral hiatus.

Technique: Press rotate 100–300 times.

Action: Relax tendons, relieve pain.

Indications: Torticollis, five kinds of stiffness and flaccidity.

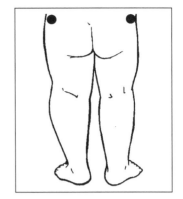

KUN LUN MOUNTAINS   KUN LUN   BL 60

Location: Depression between the external malleolus and the tendocalcaneous.

Technique: Fingernail press 5–10 times.

Action: Calm fright, relieve spasms, clear meridians and collaterals.

Indications: Convulsions, rigidity, twitching.

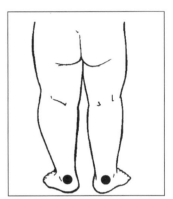

LEG THREE MILES   ZU SAN LI   ST 36

Location: Lateral aspect of the lower leg, 3 cun below and 1 cun lateral to the inferior lateral border of the patella, between the two tendons.

Technique: Fingernail press 5–10 times, then press rotate 30–50 times; *or* press rotate 100–300 times.

Action: Relieve chest, facilitate diaphragm, promote digestion, remove stagnation, eliminate spasms, relieve pain, tonify spleen, harmonize stomach, regulate middle-burner qi.

Indications: Abdominal fullness or distension, stagnant cold stomach, borborygmus, abdominal pain, convulsions, dyspnea, tachypnea, vomiting, diarrhea, weakness or atrophy of lower limbs.

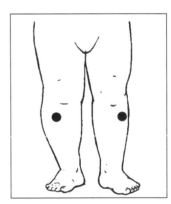

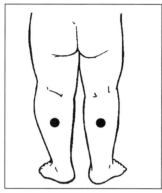

MOUNTAIN SUPPORT   CHENG SHAN   BL 57

Location: Posterior calf, directly inferior to the joining of the two heads of the gastrocnemius muscle on the posterior midline.

Technique: Fingernail press 3–5 times, then press rotate 20–30 times.

Action: Induce perspiration, relieve exterior, calm fright, expel wind.

Indications: Convulsions, twitching, tachypnea, wheezing (phlegm).

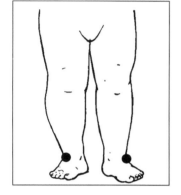

RAVINE DIVIDE   JIE XI   ST 41

Location: Top of the ankle, at the depression at the midpoint of the transverse line between two tendons, approximately at the level of the ankle-bone tip.

Technique: Fingernail press 5–10 times, then press rotate 20–50 times; or press rotate 100–200 times.

Action: Calm fright, relieve spasms, tonify spleen, harmonize stomach, stop diarrhea, remove stagnation.

Indications: Convulsions, opisthotonos, vomiting, diarrhea, motor impairment of ankle joint.

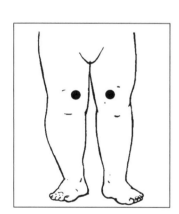

SEA OF BLOOD   XUE HAI   SP 10

Location: Medial aspect of the upper thigh, 2 cun from the superior-medial side of the patella on the bulge of the quadriceps femoris.

Technique: Press rotate 50–100 times, or fingernail press 3–5 times.

Action: Clear meridians, relax spasms.

Indications: Limb contracture, lower-limb pain and weakness.

SUBSERVIENT VISITOR   PU CAN   BL 61

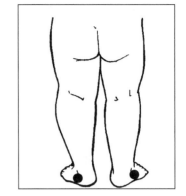

Location: Lateral ankle, behind and below the ankle bone, in the depression of the calcaneus at the junction of red and white skin (inferior to Kun Lun Mountains).

Technique: Grasp 5–10 times; *or* fingernail press 3–5 times, then press rotate 10–20 times.

Action: Calm fright, expel wind, dredge apertures, open passes.

Indications: Convulsions, fainting, cold extremities, coma.

SUSPENDED BELL   XUAN ZHONG   GB 39

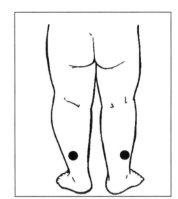

Location: 3 cun superior to the tip of the external malleolus, in the depression between the posterior border of the fibula and the muscle tendons.

Technique: Press rotate 100–300 times.

Action: Calm spasms, relax tendons and meridians.

Indications: Convulsions, atrophy of lower-extremity muscles.

THREE YIN MEETING   SAN YIN JIAO   SP 6

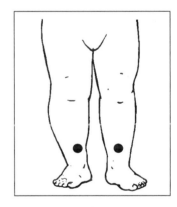

Location: Lower leg, medial side, 3 cun superior to the ankle-bone tip on the posterior edge of the tibia.

Technique: Press rotate 100–300 times; *or* push upward and downward 20–30 times, then press rotate 50–100 times; *or* fingernail press 5–10 times, then press rotate 20–30 times.

Action: Clear collaterals, activate blood, quell liver, expel wind, clear meridians, regulate lower-burner function, disperse pathogenic damp heat, readjust water passages.

Indications: Enuresis, urine retention, painful urination.

Convulsions: *Acute:* Clear by pressing (downward). *Chronic:* Tonify by pressing (upward).

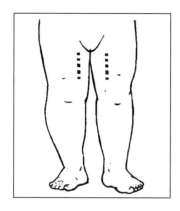

WINNOWER GATE JI MEN SP 11

Location: On the medial side of the thigh, the line from the upper border of the kneecap to the inguinal groove.

Technique: Push distal to proximal 100–300 times.

Action: Mildly diuretic.

Indications: Dysuria, yellowish urine, urine retention, watery diarrhea.

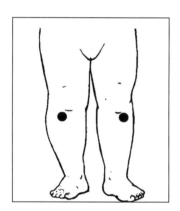

YANG MOUND SPRING YANG LING QUAN GB 34

Location: In the depression anterior and inferior to the head of the fibula.

Technique: Fingernail press 10–20 times.

Action: Relax tendons, smooth qi flow.

Indications: Convulsions, stiffness of lower extremities.

Head Region

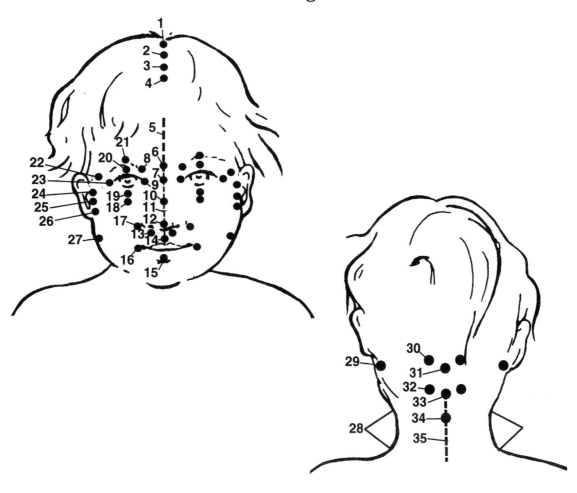

HEAD-POINT NAMES

26	Auditory Convergence	16	Earth Granary	29	Protruding Bone Behind Ear
24	Auditory Palace	20	Fish Back	23	Pupil Bone Hole
8	Bamboo Gathering	2	Fontanel Gate	15	Sauce Receptacle
3	Before Vertex	4	Fontanel Meeting	19	Tear Container
34	Between Moments	18	Four Whites	12	Tip of Nose
35	Bone of Celestial Pillar	22	Great Yang	13	Wasp Entering Cave
30	Brain Hollow	6	Hall of Authority	21	Water Palace
28	Bridge Arch	14	Human Center	17	Welcome Fragrance
9	Bright Eyes	27	Jawbone	31	Wind Mansion
5	Celestial Gate	1	Meeting of Hundreds	32	Wind Pond
11	Celestial Hearing	7	Mountain Base	10	Year Longevity
25	Ear Wind Gate	33	Mute's Gate		

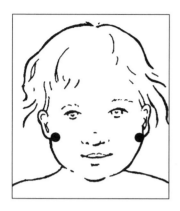

AUDITORY CONVERGENCE   TING HUI   GB 2

Location: Anterior to the intertragic notch, at the posterior border of the condyloid process of the mandible.

Technique: Press, or fingernail press 10–20 times.

Action: Expel wind cold.

Indications: Common cold, headache, earache.

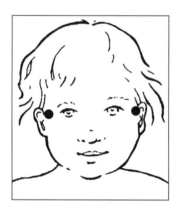

AUDITORY PALACE   TING GONG   SI 19

Location: In the jaw area, the depression when the mouth opens, anterior tragus, posterior TMJ.

Technique: Press rotate 30–50 times.

Action: Dredge and open blockages or obstructions.

Indications: Trismus, deafness, strabismus, earache.

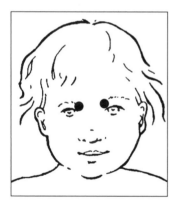

BAMBOO GATHERING   ZAN ZHU   BL 2

Location: Medial ends of the eyebrows, above the inner canthi, at the supraorbital notch.

Technique: Fingernail press bilaterally 3–7 times, then press rotate 10–20 times.

Action: Clear dizziness, relieve headache.

Indications: Headache, dizziness.

BEFORE VERTEX QIAN DING GV 21

Location: At the top-of-the-head midline, 1.5 cun anterior to Meeting of Hundreds.

Technique: Fingernail press 10–20 times, then press rotate 50–100 times; *or* press rotate 200–300 times.

Action: Tranquilize mind, relieve pain.

Indications: Headache, convulsions.

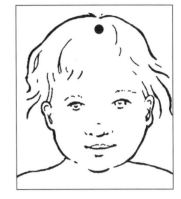

BETWEEN MOMENTS XIN JIAN

Location: Back of neck, between C-2 and C-3, and below Mute's Gate.

Technique: Pinch squeeze from four directions until red.

Action: Disperse accumulated heat, clear throat, relieve inflammation and pain.

Indications: Sore throat, acute laryngopharyngitis and tonsillitis, vocal chord edema, hoarseness.

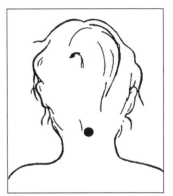

BONE OF CELESTIAL PILLAR TIAN ZHU GU

Location: Back of neck, the posterior midline from C-1 to C-7 (hairline to Great Hammer).

Technique: Push superior to inferior 100–500 times.

Action: Smooth qi flow, depress adverse rising qi, promote downward qi flow.

Indications: Occipital headache due to common cold, neck pain and stiffness, vomiting, EPI, high fever, sore throat.

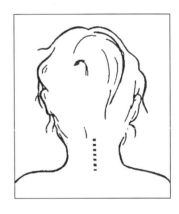

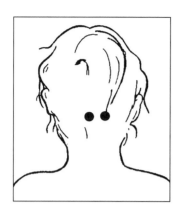

Brain Hollow   Nao kong   GB 19

Location: Back of the head, directly above Wind Pond, level with Brain's Door (GV 17), and 1.5 cun superior to the external occipital protuberance.

Technique: Fingernail press 5–8 times, then press rotate 10–20 times; *or* press rotate 50–100 times.

Action: Expel wind, relieve pain.

Indications: Headache, epilepsy.

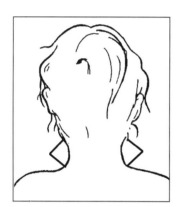

Bridge Arch   Qiao gong

Location: On the side of the neck, along the sternocleidomastoid.

Technique: Press rotate 100–500 times, *or* grasp 5–10 times, *or* rotate push 100–200 times, *or* chafe (downward) until warm.

Action: Relax tendons, activate blood.

Indications: Torticollis, stiff neck.

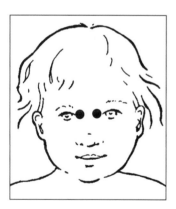

Bright Eyes   Jing ming   BL 1

Location: Near the eyes, 0.01 cun superior to the inner canthus.

Technique: Press rotate 50–100 times.

Action: Relax tendons and muscles around eyes.

Indications: Eye problems, strabismus, crossed eyes.

CELESTIAL GATE   TIAN MEN

Location: Midline of the forehead, from the mideyebrow point to the anterior hairline.

Technique: Push thumb over thumb briskly, inferior to superior, 30–50 times; *or* press 3–7 times.

Action: Expel wind, relieve exterior, open orifices, sober and tranquilize mind, calm fright, soothe nerves, relieve headache.

Indications: Convulsions, fright, palpitations, common-cold fever without perspiration, vomiting, headache, dizziness, anhidrosis, lassitude, depression, anxiety, terror, panic.

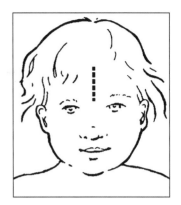

CELESTIAL HEARING   TIAN TING

Location: On the forehead, from the center of the midline (Celestial Hearing) to the depression below the lower lip (Sauce Receptacle).

Technique: Fingernail press each point 3–5 times in order.

Action: Resuscitate, relieve convulsions.

Indications: Convulsions, unconsciousness, exogenous pathogenic wind cold.

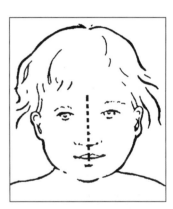

EAR WIND GATE   ER FENG MEN

Location: Near the ear, the depression with the mouth open anterior to the supratragal notch.

Technique: Rotate push both points simultaneously. *Tonify:* Forward. *Clear:* Backward.

Action: Tranquilize mind, calm fright.

Indications: Convulsions, tinnitis, deafness, toothache, earache.

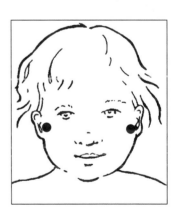

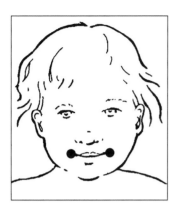

EARTH GRANARY   DI CANG   ST 4

Location: Corner of the mouth, 0.5 cun lateral.

Technique: Fingernail press 10–20 times.

Action: Expel wind, calm fright.

Indications: Deviations of mouth, convulsions.

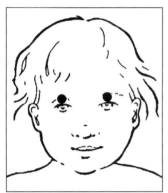

FISH BACK   YU YAO   X 5

Location: Just below the midpoint of the eyebrow, on the orbit.

Technique: Press rotate 50–100 times.

Action: Relax muscles around eye.

Indications: Eye dysfunctions, strabismus, crossed eyes.

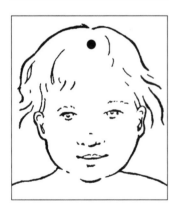

FONTANEL GATE   XIN MEN

Location: Top of the head, the depression in front of Meeting of Hundreds.

Technique: Push from anterior hairline to Fontanel Gate, then push apart to both sides 20–30 times; *or* press rotate gently 50–100 times.

Action: Expel wind, calm fright, open orifices, tranquilize mind.

Indications: Convulsions, epilepsy, twitching, dizziness, nosebleed, stuffy nose.

FONTANEL MEETING XIN HUI GV 22

Location: Midline on top of the head, 2 cun posterior to the anterior hairline.

Technique: Push from the anterior hairline to Fontanel Meeting.

Action: Soothe nerves, resuscitate.

Indications: Convulsions, spasms, dizziness, blurred vision, nasal obstruction, rhinorrhea.

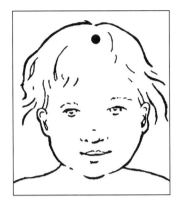

FOUR WHITES SI BAI ST 2

Location: Near the eye, the depression directly below the pupil in the infraorbital foramen.

Technique: Press rotate 100–300 times.

Action: Relax muscles, relieve pain and red eyes.

Indications: Eye problems, strabismus, crossed eyes.

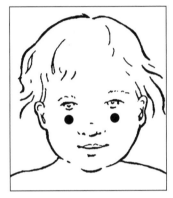

GREAT YANG TAI YANG X 1

Location: The depression at the lateral end of the eyebrows.

Technique: Rotate push 20–50 times. *Tonify:* Forward. *Clear:* Backward.

Action: Expel wind, clear heat, open orifices, calm fright.

Indications: Convulsions, fever, vexation, restlessness, common cold without perspiration, headache, eye pain, exogenous headache.

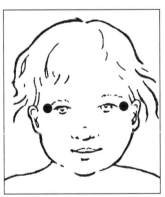

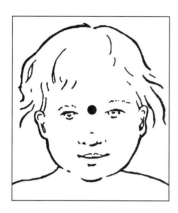

HALL OF AUTHORITY YIN TANG X 2

Location: On the forehead, the midpoint between the medial ends of the eyebrows.

Technique: Press rotate 30–50 times, *or* fingernail press 5–10 times then press rotate 20–30 times, *or* push 20–30 times.

Action: Open orifices, refresh mind, resuscitate, stop twitching.

Indications: Convulsions, epilepsy, strabismus, stuffy nose, nasal discharge.

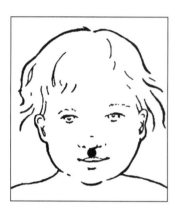

HUMAN CENTER REN ZHONG GV 26

Location: Midline of the upper lip, slightly above the midpoint.

Technique: Fingernail press 5–10 times, then press rotate 20–30 times.

Action: Calm fright, stop convulsions, open orifices, resuscitate, refresh mind, improve eyesight.

Indications: Convulsions, epilepsy, lip tic, speech impairments, jaundice, edema, spasm due to high fever.

First aid: For convulsions or spasms with high fever, fingernail press Human Center, Ten Kings, Old Dragon.

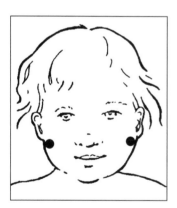

JAWBONE JIA CHE ST 6

Location: On the jaw, 1 cun anterior and superior to the annulus mandible, in the lower angle of the mandible.

Technique: Fingernail press 5–10 times, then press rotate 30–50 times; *or* press 5 times, then press rotate 30 times.

Action: Dredge and open blockages or obstructions.

Indications: Trismus, eye and mouth deviations.

MEETING OF HUNDREDS BAI HUI GV 20

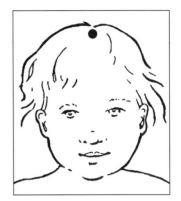

Location: Top of the head, the point where perpendicular lines from the tips of the ears intersect the midline.

Technique: Press rotate 100–300 times; *or* fingernail press 5 times, then press rotate 30–50 times; *or* press 3–7 times, then press rotate 30–50 times.

Action: Lift sunken yang and qi, ease mind, calm fright, open apertures, improve eyesight, soothe nerves, tonify vital qi.

Indications:* Convulsions, epilepsy, headache, dizziness, diarrhea, enuresis, blurred vision, nasal obstruction, prolapsed rectum, restlessness, crying, irritability, insomnia.

MOUNTAIN BASE SHAN GEN

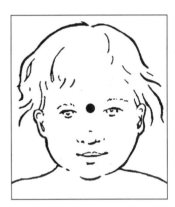

Location: Above the bridge of the nose at the midpoint between the eyebrows.

Technique:†Fingernail press 5–10 times, then press rotate 10–20 times.

Action: Reduce fever, stop convulsions, dredge passes, open orifices.

Indications: Convulsions, twitching.

MUTE'S GATE YA MEN GV 15

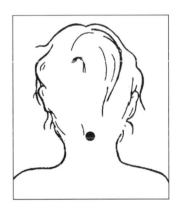

Location: 0.5 cun above the posterior hairline, in the depression inferior to the first cervical vertebra.

Technique: Fingernail press 10–20 times, *or* press rotate 100–500 times.

Action: Relieve throat.

Indications: Hoarseness, sore throat.

---

* Contraindications: Nausea, vomiting.

† Mountain Base is used more often for assessment than treatment. See chapter 5.

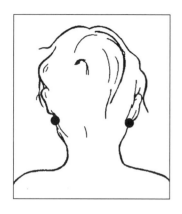

PROTRUDING BONE BEHIND EAR   ER HOU

Location: Behind the ear, the depression at the hairline posterior to the mastoid process.

Technique: Rotate push. *Tonify:* Forward 20–30 times. *Clear:* Backward 20–30 times. *Or* press rotate 20–50 times.

Action: Clear heat, expel wind, calm fright, ease mind, remove listlessness.

Indications: Headache, twitching, convulsions, vexation, restlessness, common cold, fever.

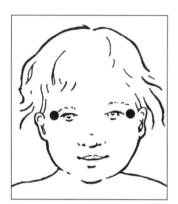

PUPIL BONE HOLE   TONG ZI LIAO   GB 1

Location: Near the eyes, 0.5 cun lateral to the outer canthus, the depression on the lateral edge of the orbit.

Technique: Press rotate 30–50 times; *or* fingernail press 3–5 times, then press rotate 20–30 times.

Action: Clear heat, calm fright, expel wind.

Indications: Convulsions, eye pain, conjunctivitis.

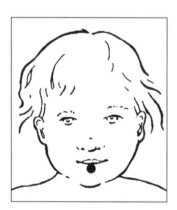

SAUCE RECEPTACLE   CHENG JIANG   CV 24

Location: The depression inferior to the lower lip.

Technique: Fingernail press 5–10 times, then press rotate 10–20 times.

Action: Tranquilize mind, calm fright, open orifices.

Indications: Convulsions, twitching, ulcerative gingivitis, diabetes, eye or mouth deviations, sudden aphonia.

TEAR CONTAINER   CHENG QI   ST 1

Location: Near the eye, directly below the pupil, between the eyeball and the infraorbital ridge.

Technique: Press rotate 50–100 times.

Action: Relax muscles and tendons around eye.

Indications: Eye muscle problems, strabismus, crossed eyes.

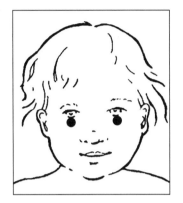

TIP OF NOSE   ZHUN TOU   GV 25

Location: Tip of the nose.

Technique: Fingernail press 5–10 times, then press rotate 10–20 times.

Action: Reduce fever, stop convulsions, dredge passes, open orifices.

Indications: Convulsions, twitching.

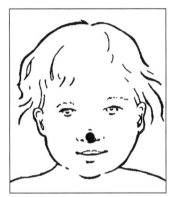

WASP ENTERING CAVE   HUANG FENG RU DONG

Location: Nostrils.

Technique: Press rotate 20–30 times.

Action: Induce perspiration, disperse pathogens from exterior, reduce fever, ventilate vital qi.

Indications: Common cold, fever, nasal obstruction.

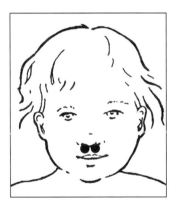

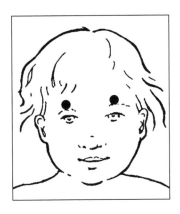

WATER PALACE KAN GONG

Location: 1 cun above the eyebrow, in a vertical line with the pupil.

Technique: Push 20–30 times, following the eyebrows, with pressure from medial to lateral only; *or* fingernail press 1 time, then push 20–30 times.

Action: Expel wind, disperse cold, open orifices, improve eyesight, induce perspiration, disperse pathogens from exterior, relieve headache.

Indications: Exogenous fever, convulsions, headache, eye redness and pain.

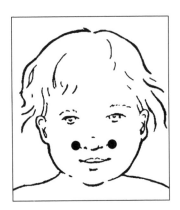

WELCOME FRAGRANCE YING XIANG LI 20

Location: 0.5 cun lateral to the side of the ala nasi in the nasolabila groove.

Technique: Fingernail press 5–10 times, then press rotate 20–40 times.

Action: Open orifices, activate collaterals.

Indications: Eye or mouth deviations, stuffy nose, nasal discharge.

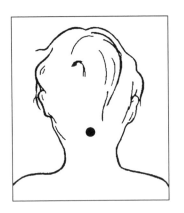

WIND MANSION FENG FU GV 16

Location: 1 cun superior to the posterior hairline, directly inferior to the external occipital protuberance.

Technique: Fingernail press 10–20 times.

Action: Relieve throat.

Indications: Hoarseness, sore throat.

Wind Pond　Feng Qi　GB 20

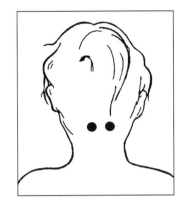

Location: Back of the head, below the base of the skull, in the depression between the sternocleidomastoid and the trapezius.

Technique: Grasp 10–20 times and simultaneously fingernail press 10–20 times, *or* press rotate 30–50 times.

Action: Induce perspiration, relieve exterior, expel wind, improve eyesight, disperse heat, expel wind cold.

Indications: Neck pain and stiffness, headache, dizziness, fever without perspiration.

Year Longevity　Nian shou

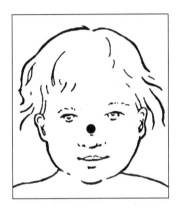

Location: On the nose, between Mountain Base and Tip of Nose.

Technique: Fingernail press 3–5 times, then press rotate 10–20 times.

Action: Dredge and open blockages and obstructions, expel wind, calm fright.

Indications: Nasal cavity dryness, stuffy nose, convulsions.

All Regions
氣

Painful Point　Ah shi (Tian ying)

Location: Any point on the body that produces a painful sensation when pressed.

Technique: Press 50–100 times, *or* press rotate 100–500 times.

Action: Disperse stagnation, relieve pain, promote flow of qi and blood.

Indications: Pain.

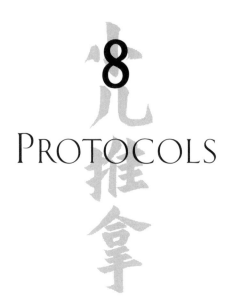

8

PROTOCOLS

THE FORMULATION OF AN INDIVIDUALIZED treatment for each child is one of the outstanding features of Chinese pediatric massage. Chinese medicine is based on using a detailed assessment to select the correct components of a treatment plan. Pediatric massage is no different.

This chapter provides a collection of treatment protocols for more than sixty different conditions. They are edited versions of protocols found in the primary sources listed in the bibliography, combined with clinical experience in both China and the United States. This is not an exhaustive list; nor does it cover all the possible variations within each condition. Instead, these protocols give general guidelines and suggestions as to how a particular pattern of disharmony might be treated. In addition, I offer examples of how different practitioners have approached patterns commonly seen in children. Still, no book can provide an accurate treatment protocol for a living, breathing, changing child.

The protocols here are not sacred, nor are they etched in stone. They are meant to be adapted, changed, and reconstructed to fit each clinical picture. Initially, you may find it helpful to learn from colleagues and their writings by using certain basic directions as guides through a treatment. Once you have internalized the material, you can create a treatment plan for each child based on your own experience.

Like acupuncture point and herb selection, the development of a pediatric massage treatment plan is a very individualized process—one that each practitioner approaches differently. A dozen practitioners could all treat the same child with a dozen different treatment plans and all be effective. This is normal and should not be considered unscientific or viewed skeptically. Many combinations of points and techniques overlap; it is possible to achieve the same results using different methods. On closer inspection, however, you will usually find that the selections of points or techniques differ only in minor ways.

For all practitioners the formulation of a treatment plan follows the assessment and analysis of the pattern of disharmony. This leads directly to the treatment principles, which then easily translate into the necessary technique and point selection. Again, however, within this framework there are many paths to the same destination.

Order of Points

Once a treatment plan is established, it is important to prioritize the order in which you manipulate the points. Several factors are important to consider.

In general, points are grouped by region and treated in the following order: hands, arms, anterior torso, posterior torso, legs, and head. Bilateral points are usually both manipulated.

If a point is likely to cause discomfort because of its location, or a technique due to its repetitive nature, it is best to reserve it until the end of the treatment.

A very useful beginning- or end-of-treatment routine consists of push Water Palace, push Celestial Gate, and press rotate Great Yang. Together these three points act to calm the child and consolidate the benefits of the other points used in the treatment.

Massage Length
氣

The length of a massage will be determined by the number of points selected and technique repetitions necessary. In general, a massage will last from fifteen to twenty-five minutes. Remember that the techniques should be performed in a very quick, brisk manner.

Massage Frequency
氣

The frequency of treatment depends on the severity and type of condition. The following are general guidelines.

Acute conditions: Daily
Severe conditions: Twice daily
Chronic or deficient conditions: Every other day

It is clearly a good idea to teach parents how to treat a few simple points daily at home.

The number of treatments necessary for a given condition will also vary according to its severity as well as your own skill in assessment, point selection, and technique. An acute condition will usually resolve in one to three treatments. A chronic condition may require ten to twenty treatments over a period of six to eight months. A more stubborn condition could take longer. Other factors, such as home massage, diet, and herbal therapy, will have a significant impact on the course of treatment. There is no magic formula that will guarantee results. A skilled practitioner will take into account the severity of the condition and the child's energetic capacity. You must also observe each treatment's effects in an ongoing process of evaluation. See chapter 9, Case Histories, for examples of course of treatments and frequency.

Protocol Arrangement
氣

Protocols in the chapter are organized in the following format:

Title
Western medical description
TCM perspective
TCM differentiation
Base protocol
Variations
Massage medium

Titles are the common names for given conditions. Western medical descriptions are self-explanatory. The TCM perspective translates the Western information into corresponding TCM terminology. Where relevant, the TCM description is differentiated by patterns of disharmony; these are general descriptions, signs, and symptoms, and may not include every possibility.

The base protocols are the common techniques and points for the differentiated assessments. I have emphasized basic points and single techniques here. Accomplished practitioners may expand these protocols with other points and multiple techniques.

The variations give additions or deletions that you may wish to make to the base protocol based on the child's specific condition.

Sesame oil is the standard massage medium for most conditions. Cool or cold water is the easiest medium for hot or excess conditions. Other massage mediums are listed with some of the variations. These are optional and are not required for each condition. See appendix F for more information on massage mediums.

ABDOMINAL DISTENSION

Description: Abdominal stretching or inflation in a convex shape.

TCM perspective: Attack of exogenous pathogens, spleen-function deficiency, improper diet.

TCM DIFFERENTIATION

Excess: Food stasis, dyspepsia, hot abdomen, nausea, foul gas, restless sleep, sallow complexion, red lips.

Tongue: Yellow coating.

Pulse: Rapid and full.

IFV: Red or deep red.

Cold: Pale complexion, cyanotic lips, cold limbs, weariness, dyspnea, desires warmth.

Tongue: Pale with a white coating.

Pulse: Deep and slow.

IFV: Pale red.

Heat: Fever, constipation, fretfulness, thirst, foul stool, deep-colored urine.

Tongue: Red with a yellow coating.

Pulse: Slippery and rapid.

IFV: Purplish.

Deficiency: Feeble digestion or elimination, sallow complexion, emaciation, cold limbs, listlessness, loose stool.

Tongue: Pale.

Pulse: Deep, thready, and stringy.

IFV: Pale red.

BASE PROTOCOL

Press rotate Spleen Meridian

Rotate push Inner Eight Symbols

Push (clear) Small Intestine Meridian

Push Below Ribs

Rotate push Abdomen

Press rotate Bubbling Spring

Press rotate Ravine Divide

Press rotate Leg Three Miles

VARIATIONS

WITH EXCESS ADD:

Push Four Transverse Lines

Push Water of Galaxy

WITH COLD ADD:

Push Three Passes

Push, then press rotate Four Transverse Lines

Press rotate External Palace of Labor

WITH HEAT ADD:

Push (clear) Large Intestine Meridian

Push (clear) Stomach Meridian

Press rotate Union Valley

Press Wood Gate

Push Water of Galaxy

Medium: Cool water

WITH DEFICIENCY ADD:

Press rotate Two Horses

Press rotate External Palace of Labor

Press rotate Kidney Meridian

Push Three Passes

ABDOMINAL PAIN

Description: Pain originating in the abdomen, possibly due to impeded function of abdominal organs.

TCM perspective: Attack of exogenous cold, improper diet, congenital deficiency, deficient and cold stomach/spleen due to prolonged illness, summer damp heat stagnation in stomach/spleen.

TCM DIFFERENTIATION

Cold: Sudden onset, pale complexion, cyanotic lips, soft abdomen, loose stool, clear urine, cold sweat on forehead, cold limbs, vomiting, diarrhea, desires warmth.

Tongue: Pale with a thin white coating.

Pulse: Tense and deep.

IFV: Red.

Cold and deficiency: Protracted, continuous pain; temporary relief after eating; aggravated with hunger; glossy pale complexion; emaciation; weariness; feebleness; cold limbs; loose stool; clear, copious urine; desires warmth.

Tongue: Pale with a white coating.

Pulse: Slow and feeble.

IFV: Pale red.

Food retention: Foul breath, belching, nausea, vomiting, foul stool.

Tongue: Red with a thick, greasy coating.

Pulse: Stringy and slippery.

IFV: Purple and stagnant.

Blood stasis and/or qi stagnation: Fixed, stabbing abdominal pain that is worse at night; dull-colored lips.

Tongue: Purple spotted.

Pulse: Deep and uneven or stringy and slippery.

IFV: Purplish.

Summer heat: Recurrent abdominal pain, hot abdomen, dry stool, deep-colored urine, thirst, large intake of water.

Tongue: Red with a yellow coating.

Pulse: Rapid.

IFV: Purple.

Base Protocol

Press rotate Spleen Meridian

Push Three Passes

Rotate push Inner Eight Symbols

Press rotate One Nestful Wind

Push Below Ribs

Rotate push Abdomen

Press rotate Bubbling Spring

Press rotate Ravine Divide

Press rotate Leg Three Miles

Push Water Palace

Press rotate Great Yang (lightly)

Variations

With cold ADD:

Increased repetitions of push Three Passes

Press rotate External Palace of Labor

Press rotate Spinal Column

Medium: Ginger or scallion decoction

With cold and deficiency ADD:

Push, then press rotate Four Transverse Lines

Press rotate Two Horses

Press rotate along both sides of Spinal Column, especially Spleen Back Point, Stomach Back Point, and Kidney Back Point

Medium: Ginger or scallion decoction

With food retention ADD:

Push (clear) Stomach Meridian

Press Wood Gate

Push (clear) Large Intestine Meridian

Medium: Chinese hawthorn decoction

With blood stasis and/or qi stagnation ADD:

Press rotate any painful point on abdomen

Press rotate Lesser Sea

Swift-shifting press

WITH SUMMER HEAT DELETE:

Push Three Passes

AND ADD:

Push (clear) Liver Meridian

Push Water of Galaxy

Push Fish for Moon Under Water

Medium: Cold water

ASTHMA

Description: Dyspnea accompanied by wheezing caused by a spasming of the bronchial tubes or swelling of the mucous membranes.

TCM perspective: Congenital deficiency, weak constitution, attack of exogenous pathogens; chronic asthma weakens lung, spleen, and kidney with accumulated damp and phlegm in respiratory tract and body.

TCM DIFFERENTIATION

Heat: Red complexion, thirst, sticky yellow phlegm, perspiration, deep-colored urine, constipation.

Tongue: Thin yellow or greasy yellow coating.

Pulse: Slippery and rapid.

IFV: Deep red or purple.

Cold: Emaciation, cold limbs, glossy pale complexion, lung phlegm that is dilute and white or clear, dilute nasal discharge, clear urine, loose stool.

Tongue: Thin white or greasy white coating.

Pulse: Superficial and slippery or soft, floating, and rapid.

IFV: Pale red.

Kidney deficiency: Dizzy, night sweats, lower back pain, oliguria with clear urine, aversion to cold, poor appetite, loose stool.

Tongue: Pale.

Pulse: Deep and weak.

IFV: Deep and pale.

Lung deficiency: Cough, weak voice, daytime perspiration, infrequent speaking, aversion to cold, white complexion.

Tongue: Pale or normal.

Pulse: Empty.

IFV: Pale.

BASE PROTOCOL

Push (clear) Lung Meridian

Press rotate Palmar Small Transverse Line

Fingernail press Vim Tranquillity

Rotate push Inner Eight Symbols

Push apart Chest Center

Push Celestial Chimney (downward)

Press rotate Celestial Chimney

Press rotate Calm Breath

Press rotate Spleen Back Point

Press rotate Lung Back Point

Push apart Scapula

VARIATIONS

WITH PHLEGM ADD:

Press rotate Snail Shell

Press rotate Bountiful Bulge

WITH HEAT ADD:

Push, and press rotate Five Digital Joints

Push Water of Galaxy

WITH COLD ADD:

Press rotate Kidney Meridian

Push Three Passes

Press rotate External Palace of Labor

WITH KIDNEY DEFICIENCY ADD:

Press rotate Two Horses

Push Three Passes

Press rotate Kidney Meridian

Press rotate Kidney Back Point

Rotate push Abdomen

Medium: Ginger decoction

WITH LUNG DEFICIENCY DELETE:

Push (clear) Lung Meridian

AND ADD:

Press rotate Lung Meridian

Push Three Passes

Press rotate Kidney Meridian

BLEEDING FROM NOSE OR GUMS, NONTRAUMATIC

Description: Bleeding without a known traumatic origin.

TCM perspective: Deficient lung/stomach heat, deficient liver/kidney yin fire, deficient qi and blood.

TCM DIFFERENTIATION

Lung heat: Dry, bleeding nasal cavity; bright red blood; irritated cough with little phlegm; fever; dry mouth.

Tongue: Red with a yellow coating.

Pulse: Rapid.

IFV: Deep red.

Stomach heat: Bad breath, dry nasal cavity, nasal and gum bleeding, bright red blood, thirst, vexation, chest oppression, dry stool, yellow urine.

Tongue: Red with a yellow coating.

Pulse: Full and rapid.

IFV: Purple-red.

Liver heat: Headache, dizziness, dry mouth, epistaxis with profuse bright red blood, deep-colored urine.

Tongue: Red with a yellow coating.

Pulse: Stringy and rapid.

IFV: Purple and stagnant.

Deficiency fire: Toothache, tinnitus, dizziness, dry throat, bleeding gums with pale red blood.

Tongue: Red.

Pulse: Thready and rapid.

IFV: Pale red

Qi deficiency: Glossy pale complexion, listlessness, feebleness, pale lips.

    Tongue: Pale.

    Pulse: Thready and weak.

    IFV: Pale red.

BASE PROTOCOL

Push Wood Gate

Push Water of Galaxy

Push Celestial Gate

VARIATIONS

WITH LUNG HEAT ADD:

Press rotate Kidney Meridian

Push (clear) Lung Meridian

Push Six Hollow Bowels

Press rotate Symmetric Upright

Press rotate Yang Marsh

Medium: Cold water

WITH STOMACH HEAT ADD:

Push (clear) Stomach Meridian

Push (clear) Small Intestine Meridian

Rotate push Inner Eight Symbols

Push Bone of Seven Segments (downward)

Press rotate Leg Three Miles

Medium: Cold water

WITH LIVER HEAT ADD:

Push Liver Meridian back and forth

Press rotate Two Horses

Press rotate Kidney Meridian

Push (clear) Stomach Meridian

Medium: Cold water

WITH DEFICIENCY FIRE ADD:

Press rotate Two Horses

Press rotate Small Celestial Center

Press rotate Kidney Meridian

Press rotate Spleen Meridian

Rotate push Inner Eight Symbols

Push Fish for Moon Under Water

Medium: Cold water

WITH QI DEFICIENCY DELETE:

Push Wood Gate

Push Water of Galaxy

AND ADD:

Press rotate Spleen Meridian

Press rotate Kidney Meridian

Press rotate Lung Meridian

Press rotate Leg Three Miles

Push Three Passes

Spinal pinch pull

Press rotate Meeting of Hundreds

Medium: Ginger juice

BRONCHITIS, ACUTE

Description: Short, severe course of bronchial tube inflammation.

TCM perspective: External invasion of wind accompanied by cold or heat, lung damp phlegm accumulation.

TCM DIFFERENTIATION

Wind cold: Aversion to wind and cold, no sweating, slight fever, stuffy nose, clear mucus, sneezing.

Tongue: Thin with a white coating.

Pulse: Floating and tight.

IFV: Red and superficial.

Wind or heat: Fever, sweating, thick yellow mucus, sore throat, cough.

Tongue: Thin white coating with red tip.

Pulse: Fast and floating.

IFV: Deep red.

Lung phlegm heat accumulation: Cough, difficult breathing, white or yellow mucus, fever.

Tongue: Thick white coating with red tip and sides.

Pulse: Slippery and rapid.

IFV: Deep red or purple.

BASE PROTOCOL

Push (clear) Lung Meridian

Press rotate Spleen Meridian

Fingernail press, then press rotate Five Digital Joints

Push Three Passes

Press rotate, then push apart Chest Center

Push Scapula

Press rotate Calm Breath

Press rotate Bubbling Spring

Push Water Palace

VARIATIONS

WITH COLD ADD:

Press rotate External Palace of Labor

Push Celestial Gate

WITH HEAT ADD:

Press rotate Inner Palace of Labor

Push Water of Galaxy

WITH LUNG PHLEGM HEAT ADD:

Press rotate Outside Nipple

Push Water of Galaxy

Push Celestial Chimney

BRONCHITIS, CHRONIC

Description: Long duration (three months to two years) of continuous low-grade bronchial tube infection.

TCM perspective: Empty lung qi. (*Note*: A progressively deteriorating case of bronchitis may lead to lung-kidney emptiness and/or spleen emptiness. See the asthma protocol on page 121.)

TCM DIFFERENTIATION

Empty lung qi: Weak cough with thin white mucus, shortness of breath, wheezing, pale complexion, tires easily.

Tongue: White body with a thin white coating.

Pulse: Deep and weak.

IFV: Deep and pale red.

BASE PROTOCOL

Press rotate Lung Meridian

Press rotate Two Horses

Press rotate Spleen Meridian

Press rotate Kidney Meridian

Push Three Passes

Push apart Chest Center

Rotate push Abdomen

Press rotate Calm Breath

Press rotate Lung Back Point

Push apart Scapula

Press rotate Spinal Column, especially Lung and Kidney Back Points

Press rotate Bubbling Spring

Press rotate Meeting of Hundreds

CHICKEN POX

Description: Acute viral disease with headache, fever, and malaise followed by red dotlike eruptions.

TCM perspective: Attack of seasonal pathogens and accumulated damp heat.

TCM DIFFERENTIATION

Mild case: Fever, headache, cough, poor appetite, stuffy nose, nasal discharge, oval red eruptions with clear pus, sparse distribution, slight itching.

Tongue: Red with a thin white or yellow coating.

Pulse: Superficial and rapid.

IFV: Bright red.

Severe case: Strong fever; red complexion and lips; mouth ulcers; listlessness, dim purple eruptions with turbid pus that are large, dense, and very itchy; deep-colored urine; dry stool.

Tongue: Red with a yellow coating

Pulse: Rapid and full or slippery.

IFV: Purplish red.

BASE PROTOCOL: MILD CASE

Push (clear) Lung Meridian

Press rotate Kidney Meridian

Press rotate Small Celestial Center

Press rotate One Nestful Wind

Rotate push Inner Eight Symbols

Push Wood Gate

Push Water of Galaxy

Press rotate Bubbling Spring

Medium: Scallion decoction

BASE PROTOCOL: SEVERE CASE

Press rotate Spleen Meridian

Push apart Large Transverse Line

Press rotate Inner Palace of Labor

Press rotate Two Horses

Push Six Hollow Bowels

Push Three Passes

VARIATIONS: MILD OR SEVERE CASE

WHEN NO NEW ERUPTIONS OCCUR DELETE:

Press rotate Spleen Meridian

Push Three Passes

Medium: Warm water or egg white

WITH HIGH FEVER (OVER 100°F/38°C) DELETE:

Press rotate Spleen Meridian

Push Three Passes

AND ADD:

Push (clear) Stomach Meridian

Lash Horse to Cross Galaxy

WITH COUGH ADD:

Push (clear) Liver Meridian

Push apart Chest Center

Press Celestial Chimney

Press rotate Breast Root

WITH LOW FEVER ADD:

Push (clear) Stomach Meridian

Push (clear) Lung Meridian

Push Water of Galaxy

WITH ABDOMINAL PAIN ADD:

Push Below Ribs

Rotate push Abdomen

WITH VOMITING ADD:

Push Large Transverse Line to Wood Gate

Press rotate Union Valley

Press rotate Leg Three Miles

COLIC

Description: *Infantile colic* is a very general term used to describe a wide range of symptoms occurring in children from birth to several years old. While the symptoms may vary, in general they all relate to some degree of pain, discomfort, restlessness, or crying, usually with no apparent cause.

TCM perspective: Two major aspects of colic may be involved in an individual child. The digestive system is considered inherently weak in infants and frequently may cause colic symptoms. Also, restlessness, anxiety, and fearful sleep or waking can be explained as the child's energy not being settled or grounded properly in the body. An unusual, frightening experience may be a source of colic symptoms as well. In the United States colic is usually related to spleen deficiency. See appendix F for an external herbal colic remedy.

TCM DIFFERENTIATION

Spleen deficiency: Feeding-, digestion-, elimination-related symptoms; loose stool; pale lips; constant low, feeble cry; poor or inconsistent appetite. Tongue: Pale.

Pulse: Slow.

IFV: Pale red.

Heart fire: Restlessness, aversion to light or heat, sharp and loud crying, red complexion and lips, hot body, constipation.

Tongue: Red or red tipped.

Pulse: Rapid.

IFV: Dark red or purple.

Fright: Sudden crying, sudden bluish or white complexion of lips, easily alarmed.

Tongue: Normal or red.

Pulse: Abrupt and rapid.

IFV: Dark or black.

BASE PROTOCOL

Press rotate Spleen Meridian

Press rotate Wood Gate

Press rotate One Nestful Wind

Push Three Passes

Rotate push Abdomen

Spinal pinch pull

Press rotate Bubbling Spring

Press rotate Ravine Divide

Press rotate Leg Three Miles

Push Water Palace

Push Celestial Gate

Press rotate Great Yang

VARIATIONS

WITH SPLEEN DEFICIENCY ADD:

Rotate push Inner Eight Symbols

Press rotate External Palace of Labor

WITH HEART FIRE ADD:

Push Water of Galaxy

Push apart Large Transverse Line

WITH FRIGHT ADD:

Press rotate Inner Palace of Labor

Press rotate Small Celestial Center

COMMON COLD

Description: *Common cold* is a general term for inflammation of the respiratory mucous membranes. It may include congestion, watery discharge, sneezing, tearing.

TCM perspective: Attack of exogenous pathogens, weak defensive qi, weather or seasonal changes.

TCM Differentiation

Wind cold: Light or no fever, headache, no perspiration, dilute nasal discharge, unproductive cough.

Tongue: Pale red with a thin white coating.

Pulse: Tense and superficial.

IFV: Superficial and red.

Wind heat: Fever, turbid nasal discharge, productive cough with yellow phlegm, throat pain, swelling, poor appetite, yellowish red urine, constipation.

Tongue: Red with a yellow coating.

Pulse: Superficial and rapid.

IFV: Deep red.

Base Protocol

Push (clear) Lung Meridian

Grasp Wind Pond

Push Celestial Gate

Rotate push Great Yang (lightly)

Push Water Palace

Variations

With runny nose ADD:

Press rotate Welcome Fragrance

Press rotate Wasp Entering Cave

With wind cold ADD:

Push Three Passes

Press rotate Two Leaf Doors

TO INDUCE SWEAT ADD:

Press rotate Outer Pass

Press rotate Broken Sequence

Grasp Great Hammer

Medium: Scallion and ginger decoction

WITH WIND OR HEAT ADD:

Push Water of Galaxy

Press rotate One Nestful Wind

Press rotate Small Celestial Center

Medium: Peppermint decoction

WITH FEVER ADD:

Push Water of Galaxy

Push, then press rotate Five Digital Joints

Increased repetitions of push Celestial Gate

Increased repetitions of push Water Palace, alternating fast and slow, superficial
and deep

Push Spinal Column (downward)

Rotate push Inner Palace of Labor

WITH COUGH ADD:

Rotate push Inner Eight Symbols

Push apart Chest Center

Push Celestial Chimney (downward)

WITH PHLEGM ADD:

Push Wood Gate

Push apart Large Transverse Line

Press rotate Breast Root

Press rotate Lung Back Point

TO STRENGTHEN AFTER COLD ADD:

Rotate push Inner Eight Symbols

Push Three Passes

Press rotate Spleen Back Point

Spinal pinch pull (upward)

Press rotate Leg Three Miles

Rotate push Abdomen

CONSTIPATION

Description: Sluggish, infrequent, or difficult bowel movements, with passage of hard and/or dry stool.

TCM perspective: Excess or deficiency with a congenital basis or due to lung, spleen, or stomach/spleen patterns.

TCM DIFFERENTIATION

Excess stagnant heat: Yang-dominant constitution; overeating of fatty, rich foods; dry stool; thirst; red complexion; fever; belching; deep-colored urine; desires liquids.

Tongue: Pale red.

Pulse: Rapid and full.

IFV: Pale, stagnant, and purple.

Excess exogenous heat: Dry stool; abdominal distension; vomiting; fretful, painful, difficult bowel movements followed by relief; red complexion and lips.

Tongue: Red with a thin yellow coating.

Pulse: Slippery and rapid.

IFV: Purple and stagnant.

Deficient congenital qi: Emaciation; thin build; glossy pale complexion; listlessness; feeble breath; low crying sounds; painful, difficult bowel movements; pale red lips.

Tongue: Pale red.

Pulse: Weak and deep.

IFV: Pale and stagnant.

Spleen/lung deficiency: Poor appetite, weariness, sallow complexion, emaciation.

Tongue: Pale with little coating.

Pulse: Thready and rapid.

IFV: Pale, red, deep, and stagnant.

BASE PROTOCOL

    Push (clear) Large Intestine Meridian

    Rotate push Inner Eight Symbols

    Press rotate Spleen Meridian

    Push Below Ribs

    Rotate push Abdomen

    Push Bone of Seven Segments (downward)

    Press rotate Tortoise Tail

    Press rotate Leg Three Miles

    Push Water Palace

    Press rotate Great Yang (lightly)

VARIATIONS

WITH EXCESS STAGNANT HEAT ADD:

Press rotate Union Valley

Push Six Hollow Bowels

Push (clear) Stomach Meridian

Medium: Relagar powder in sesame oil

WITH EXCESS EXOGENOUS HEAT ADD:

Rotate push Outer Eight Symbols

Push Water of Galaxy

Press rotate Arm Yang Pool

WITH DEFICIENT CONGENITAL QI ADD:

Press rotate Kidney Summit

Press rotate Two Horses

Rub palms together, then cover Elixir Field and Life Gate

WITH SPLEEN/LUNG DEFICIENCY ADD:

Press rotate Lung Meridian

Press rotate Lung Back Point

Press rotate Spleen Back Point

Grasp Shoulder Well

Description: A short-term, periodic, and sudden attack of involuntary muscle contractions and relaxations.

TCM perspective: There are two major differentiations: exogenous attack and internal stagnation. The former involves exogenous seasonal pathogens and accumulated endogenous heat. Internal stagnation involves excess internal heat that creates liver wind, pericardium fire from food, and/or phlegm stasis. Fright may create liver wind.

TCM DIFFERENTIATION: EXOGENOUS ATTACK

Wind: Fever, headache, cough, stuffy nose, nasal discharge, red throat, swelling and pain, fretfulness, convulsions, possible unconsciousness.

Tongue: Thin and yellow coating.

Pulse: Superficial and rapid.

IFV: Red.

Summer heat: Fever, headache, chest oppression, nausea, vomiting, listlessness, drowsiness, stiff neck, convulsions.

Tongue: Thin and greasy yellow coating.

Pulse: Slippery and rapid.

IFV: Deep red.

Epidemic pathogens: Sudden fever, coma, fretfulness, restlessness, thirst, dry throat, delirium, convulsions, twitching.

Tongue: Deep red or crimson with a dry yellow coating.

Pulse: Full, rapid, and stringy.

IFV: Deep red.

Heat invading pericardium and ying qi: Coma; twitching limbs; hot torso, palms, or soles; cold limbs; skin eruptions.

Tongue: Crimson.

Pulse: Stringy, thready, and rapid.

IFV: Purplish black.

BASE PROTOCOL: EXOGENOUS ATTACK

Pound Small Celestial Center

Fingernail press Five Digital Joints

Fingernail press Sweet Load

Push apart Large Transverse Line

Push Water of Galaxy

Fingernail press Central Hub

Fingernail press Human Center

Press rotate Fontanel Meeting

Press rotate Subservient Visitor

VARIATIONS

WITH WIND ADD:

Fingernail press Ten Kings

Push (clear) Lung Meridian

Push Celestial Gate

WITH SUMMER HEAT ADD:

Fingernail press One Nestful Wind

Grasp Mountain Support

Grasp Broken Sequence

WITH EPIDEMIC PATHOGENS ADD:

Press rotate Two Leaf Doors

Press rotate Kidney Meridian

Rotate push Inner Eight Symbols

Medium: Cold water

WITH HEAT INVADING PERICARDIUM AND YING QI ADD:

Fingernail press Hall of Authority

Fingernail press Sauce Receptacle

Push Six Hollow Bowels

Push Fish for Moon Under Water

Medium: Cold water

TCM DIFFERENTIATION: INTERNAL STAGNATION

Food obstruction: Poor appetite, sour and putrid vomit, abdominal distension and pain, constipation, fever, wheezing due to phlegm, greenish blue complexion, dull mind, convulsions, twitching.

Tongue: Pale with a yellow, dirty, greasy coating.

Pulse: Rapid.

IFV: Cyanotic.

Damp heat: High fever with chills, delirium, nausea, vomiting, abdominal distension and pain, odorous stool, stool mixed with pus and blood, coma, twitching, recurrent convulsions.

Tongue: Red with a greasy yellow coating.

Pulse: Slippery and rapid.

IFV: Dark and cyanotic.

Fright: Constitutional weakness, low or no fever, cold limbs, restless sleep, alternating red and greenish blue complexion, greenish blue stool.

Tongue: Thin coating.

Pulse: Deep.

IFV: Dark and cyanotic.

BASE PROTOCOL: INTERNAL STAGNATION

Fingernail press Small Transverse Lines

Press rotate Small Celestial Center

Press rotate Five Digital Joints

Rotate push Inner Eight Symbols

Push Water of Galaxy

VARIATIONS

WITH FOOD OBSTRUCTION ADD:

Press rotate Spleen Meridian

Push Wood Gate

Push apart Large Transverse Line

Rotate push Abdomen

Push Below Ribs

Fingernail press Leg Three Miles

WITH DAMP HEAT ADD:

Push (clear) Liver Meridian

Fingernail press Two Leaf Doors

Grasp Ghost Eye

Grasp Bend Middle

WITH FRIGHT ADD:

Fingernail press Human Center

Fingernail press Hall of Authority

Fingernail press Bubbling Spring

Press rotate Meeting of Hundreds

WITH WHEEZING ADD:

Fingernail press Bountiful Bulge

WITH HIGH FEVER ADD:

Fingernail press Ten Kings

Fingernail press Pool at the Bend

Grasp Wind Pond

CONVULSIONS, CHRONIC

Description: A long-standing condition of periodic sudden attacks of involuntary muscle contractions and relaxations.

TCM perspective: Spleen or kidney/spleen damage due to serious vomiting or diarrhea, protracted illness, kidney/liver yin depletion due to febrile diseases, spleen deficiency, wind created by yin depletion.

TCM Differentiation

Spleen yang deficiency: Listlessness, drowsiness, sleeping with eyes half closed, sallow complexion, cold limbs, edema of face and feet, twitching.

Tongue: Pale with a white coating.

Pulse: Deep and weak.

IFV: Pale and cyanotic.

Kidney/spleen yang deficiency: Listlessness, glossy pale complexion, cold sweat on forehead, cold limbs, lethargy, coma, clear and loose stool.

Tongue: Pale with a thin white coating.

Pulse: Deep and faint.

IFV: Pale red.

Liver/kidney yin depletion: Vexation, weariness, flushing, emaciation, hot palms and soles, spasms, rigid or twitching limbs, constipation.

Tongue: Red and dry with no coating.

Pulse: Deep, thready, and rapid.

IFV: Pale purple or cyanotic.

BASE PROTOCOL

Press rotate Two Horses

Press rotate, or pound Small Celestial Center

Fingernail press, then press rotate Five Digital Joints

Push Three Passes

Push apart Large Transverse Line

Rotate push Inner Eight Symbols

VARIATIONS

WITH SPLEEN YANG DEFICIENCY ADD:

Press rotate Kidney Meridian

Press rotate Spleen Meridian

Press rotate Spleen Back Point

Press rotate Stomach Back Point

WITH KIDNEY/SPLEEN YANG DEFICIENCY ADD:

Press rotate Kidney Summit

Press rotate Spleen Meridian

Press rotate Spleen Back Point

Press rotate Stomach Back Point

Press rotate Kidney Back Point

Medium: Chinese ilex oil

WITH LIVER/KIDNEY YIN DEPLETION ADD:

Push (clear) Liver Meridian

Press rotate Spleen Meridian

Press rotate One Nestful Wind

Grasp Hundreds Worms Nest

Red Phoenix Nods Head

Description: Conditions present after an attack of convulsive activity has passed.

BASE PROTOCOL

Press rotate Spleen Meridian

Press rotate Kidney Meridian

Press rotate, or pound Small Celestial Center

VARIATIONS

WITH UPPER-LIMB DISABILITY ADD:

Press rotate Great Hammer

Push Spinal Column (upward) from level of T-12 to T-1

Press rotate Spleen Back Point

Press rotate Stomach Back Point

Press affected limb

Rub roll affected limb

WITH LOWER-LIMB DISABILITY ADD:

Push along both sides of Spinal Column (downward)

Press affected limb

Rub roll affected limb

WITH STRABISMUS ADD:

Press rotate Yang Marsh

Press rotate with thumb: Fish Back, Bright Eyes, and Bamboo Gathering

Press rotate Great Yang

Press rotate Wind Pond

Grasp Shoulder Well

WITH HOARSE VOICE ADD:

Fingernail press Five Digital Joints

Fingernail press Mute's Gate

Fingernail press Wind Mansion

WITH EXCESS PHLEGM ADD:

Push Water of Galaxy

Press rotate Celestial Chimney

Rotate push Outer Eight Symbols

Push apart Chest Center

COUGH

Description: Forceful, possibly violent expiratory effort preceded by an inspiration.

TCM perspective: Attack of exogenous pathogens on lung causes adverse rising of qi; deficient spleen or lung yin qi causes phlegm.

TCM DIFFERENTIATION

Wind cold: Frequent coughing with dilute white phlegm, headache, fever, aversion to cold, no perspiration, itchy throat, aching body.

Tongue: Thin white coating.

Pulse: Tense and superficial.

IFV: Superficial and pale red.

Wind heat: Chest oppression, sticky yellow phlegm, thirst, sore throat, turbid nasal discharge, fever, headache, slight perspiration.

Tongue: Thin with a yellow coating.

Pulse: Superficial and rapid.

IFV: Superficial and deep red.

Lung heat: Sudden recurrent cough, sticky phlegm, dry throat, fever, thirst, red complexion and lips, deep-colored urine, dry stool, restlessness.

Tongue: Red without coating, deficient saliva.

Pulse: Rapid and slippery.

IFV: Deep red.

Phlegm damp: Profuse and dilute white phlegm, chest fullness, no appetite, listlessness, condition worsens at night.

Tongue: Pale with a yellowish white coating.

Pulse: Slippery.

IFV: Red-purple.

Yin deficiency: Unproductive cough or difficult-to-expectorate phlegm, itchy throat, hoarse voice, hot soles and palms, afternoon fever.

Tongue: Red with little coating.

Pulse: Rapid and thready.

IFV: Pale or light red.

Spleen/lung qi deficiency: Feeble cough with dilute white phlegm, glossy complexion, shortness of breath, low voice, aversion to cold, desires warmth.

Tongue: Pale and tender.

Pulse: Thready and feeble.

IFV: Pale or light red.

BASE PROTOCOL

Push (clear) Lung Meridian

Push, then press rotate Five Digital Joints

Rotate push Inner Eight Symbols

Push apart Chest Center

Push Celestial Chimney (downward)

Push apart Scapula

Press rotate Lung Back Point

Press Water Palace

Press rotate Great Yang

Press Celestial Gate

VARIATIONS

WITH WIND COLD ADD:

Push Three Passes

Grasp Wind Pond

Press rotate Wind Gate

Medium: Ginger juice

WITH WIND HEAT ADD:

Press rotate One Nestful Wind

Press rotate Small Celestial Center

Press rotate Lesser Marsh

Push Water of Galaxy

Medium: Peppermint decoction

WITH LUNG HEAT ADD:

Press rotate Palmar Small Transverse Line

Press rotate Two Leaf Doors

Pinch squeeze Celestial Chimney

WITH PHLEGM DAMP ADD:

Press rotate Spleen Meridian

Press rotate White Tendon

Push, then press rotate Four Transverse Lines

WITH YIN DEFICIENCY ADD:

Press rotate Kidney Meridian

Press rotate Two Horses

Press rotate Bubbling Spring

WITH SPLEEN OR LUNG QI DEFICIENCY DELETE:

Push (clear) Lung Meridian

AND ADD:

Press rotate Spleen Meridian

Press rotate Lung Meridian

Push Three Passes

Press rotate Two Horses

Press rotate Meeting of Hundreds

DELAYED FONTANEL CLOSURE

Description: Junction between cranial bones of the skull, which normally close together with unossified space by the end of first or second year after birth.

TCM perspective: Congenital deficiency, or deficiency of the spleen and kidney due to protracted illness.

BASE PROTOCOL

Press rotate Two Horses

Press rotate Kidney Meridian

Press rotate Kidney Summit

Push Six Hollow Bowels

Press rotate Meeting of Hundreds

VARIATIONS

WITH SHAKING HEAD AND CRYING ADD:

Press rotate Fish Border

Press rotate One Nestful Wind

Push Small Transverse Lines

WITH CONSTIPATION ADD:

Push (clear) Large Intestine Meridian

Rotate push Abdomen

Push Bone of Seven Segments (downward)

WITHOUT SYMPTOMS, BUT CHILD IS PALE AND EMACIATED, ADD:

Press rotate Spleen Meridian

Push Three Passes

DIABETES

Description: A metabolic disorder characterized by hypoglycemia and excessive urination due to inadequate production or utilization of insulin.

TCM perspective: Protracted lung and stomach dryness creates kidney yin depletion.

BASE PROTOCOL

Push (clear) Lung Meridian

Press rotate Two Horses

Press rotate Spleen Meridian

Press rotate External Palace of Labor

Push Six Hollow Bowels

Press rotate Yang Marsh

DIARRHEA

Description: Frequent bowel movements of loose and/or watery stool.

TCM perspective: Attack of exogenous pathogens, or immature or deficient stomach/spleen.

Diarrhea is a common condition in children due to their inherent middle-burner weakness. Occasional short periods of diarrhea may be considered normal. A mild case of diarrhea can be defined as having few symptoms or other effects on the child and lasting longer than a normal case. A severe case of diarrhea is indicated by severe symptoms over a longer time period, dehydration, and a larger impact on the other energetic functions of the child.

TCM Differentiation: Mild

Cold damp: Pale complexion and lips, no thirst, no dryness of mouth, cold aversion, cold limbs.

Tongue: White and moist coating.

Pulse: Slow.

IFV: Reddish.

Heat: Sudden onset, thirst, hot-body feeling, perspiration.

Tongue: Yellow and greasy coating.

Pulse: Smooth.

IFV: Purple.

Improper eating: Distension and pain of abdominal region, relief after bowel movement.

Tongue: Greasy.

Pulse: Slippery and rapid.

IFV: Purple.

Fragile spleen: Recurrent diarrhea, undigested food in stool, abdominal fullness, no thirst, emaciation, listlessness.

Tongue: Pale with a thin coating.

Pulse: Soft, floating, and slow; or deep and feeble.

IFV: Reddish.

Chronic: A simple case of diarrhea due to exogenous factors or temporary spleen and/or kidney deficiency that does not resolve quickly. Symptoms will vary according to energetic causes.

TCM Differentiation: Severe

Protracted: Emaciation, aversion to cold, glossy pale complexion, listlessness, cold limbs, child sleeps with eyes half closed.

Tongue: Pale and thick with a thin white coating.

Pulse: Faint and thready.

IFV: Pale.

Yin damage: Listlessness, eye orbit depression, dry skin, inelastic skin, watery yellow stool, thirst, reddened lips.

Tongue: Crimson without saliva.

Pulse: Faint and rapid.

IFV: Deep and red-purple.

Yang damage: Pale complexion, cold limbs, perspiration without fever.

    Tongue: Pale

    Pulse: Deep and thready.

    IFV: Deep and pale.

Yin/yang damage: Glossy pale complexion, sleepiness, cold limbs, sunken abdomen, crying without tears.

    Tongue: Red without coating.

    Pulse: Deep and faint.

    IFV: Deep.

Kidney deficiency: Early-morning diarrhea, calm after bowel movement, dark complexion, aversion to cold, cold limbs.

    Tongue: Pale.

    Pulse: Weak.

    IFV: Deep and pale.

BASE PROTOCOL: MILD

Press rotate Spleen Meridian

Push (clear) Small Intestine Meridian

Push Three Passes

Rotate push Inner Eight Symbols

Press rotate Celestial Pivot

Push Below Ribs

Rotate push Abdomen

Push Bone of Seven Segments (upward)

Press rotate Bubbling Spring

Press rotate Ravine Divide

Press rotate Leg Three Miles

VARIATIONS

WITH COLD DAMP ADD:

Increased repetitions of push Three Passes

Rub palms together, then cover Spirit Gate

WITH WIND ADD:

Press rotate Small Celestial Center

Press rotate One Nestful Wind

Press rotate External Palace of Labor

Medium: Warm ginger or scallion decoction

WITH HEAT DELETE:

Push Three Passes

AND ADD:

Push (clear) Large Intestine Meridian

Push Six Hollow Bowels

Push (clear) Stomach Meridian

WITH DAMP ADD:

Push Water of Galaxy

Push (clear) Wood Gate

Medium: Scute or coptis decoction

WITH IMPROPER EATING ADD:

Increased repetitions of push Below Ribs

Push (clear) Large Intestine Meridian

Grasp Abdominal Corner

Medium: Chinese hawthorn decoction

WITH FRAGILE SPLEEN ADD:

Increased repetitions of press rotate Spleen Meridian

Press rotate Kidney Meridian

Press rotate Wood Gate

Press rotate Meeting of Hundreds

Press rotate Spinal Column, emphasizing Spleen Back Point and Stomach Back Point

WITH VOMITING ADD:

Press rotate Union Valley

Press rotate Outside Nipple

WITH CHRONIC DIARRHEA (NO ABDOMINAL DISTENSION, NO IMPROPER EATING) ADD:

Push Bone of Seven Segments (upward)

Press rotate Tortoise Tail

Medium: Ginger decoction

BASE PROTOCOL: SEVERE

Press rotate Spleen Meridian

Push (clear) Small Intestine Meridian

Push Three Passes

Rotate push Inner Eight Symbols

Press rotate Celestial Pivot

Push Below Ribs

Rotate push Abdomen

Push Bone of Seven Segments (upward)

Press rotate Bubbling Spring

Press rotate Ravine Divide

Press rotate Leg Three Miles

VARIATIONS

WITH PROTRACTED DIARRHEA ADD:

Press rotate Kidney Meridian

Push apart Large Transverse Line

Press rotate Spleen Back Point

Press rotate Kidney Back Point

Press rotate Meeting of Hundreds

Medium: Ginger decoction

WITH YIN DAMAGE ADD:

Push Transport Earth to Water

Push apart Large Transverse Line

Press rotate Lung Back Point

Press rotate Heart Back Point

Press rotate Spleen Back Point

WITH YANG DAMAGE ADD:

Increased repetitions of push Three Passes

Press rotate Large Intestine Meridian

Push Transport Earth to Water

Press rotate Spleen Back Point

Press rotate Lung Back Point

Medium: Dilute ginger decoction

WITH YIN/YANG DAMAGE ADD:

Push Wood Gate to Large Transverse Line

Push apart Large Transverse Line

Press rotate Meeting of Hundreds

Press rotate Mountain Support

Medium: Dilute ginger decoction

WITH KIDNEY DEFICIENCY ADD:

Press rotate Kidney Meridian

Press rotate Two Horses

Press rotate External Palace of Labor

DIGESTION, POOR

Description: Incomplete or imperfect digestive process, lack of desire to eat. Also called indigestion, loss of appetite.

TCM perspective: Improper eating habits, congenital or postnatal stomach/spleen deficiency.

TCM DIFFERENTIATION

Spleen damp: Poor appetite, nausea, vomiting, abdominal distension, listlessness, no thirst, loose stool.

Tongue: Red with a thin, greasy yellow coating.

Pulse: Slippery, rapid, and energetic.

IFV: Purple.

Stomach/spleen deficiency: Sallow complexion, emaciation, feebleness, loose stools or frequent diarrhea.

Tongue: Pale with little coating.

Pulse: Weak and thready.

IFV: Pale red.

BASE PROTOCOL

Press rotate Spleen Meridian

Push Three Passes

Rotate push Inner Eight Symbols

Fingernail press, then press rotate Four Transverse Lines

Push Below Ribs

Rotate push Abdomen

Spinal pinch pull

Press rotate along both sides of Spinal Column, especially Spleen and Stomach
    Back Points

Press rotate Bubbling Spring

Press rotate Ravine Divide

Press rotate Leg Three Miles

VARIATIONS

WITH VOMITING ADD:

Press rotate Outside Nipple

Press rotate Union Valley

WITH SPLEEN DAMP ADD:

Push apart Large Transverse Line

Push Wood Gate

Push Water of Galaxy

Medium: Scallion or ginger decoction

WITH STOMACH OR SPLEEN DEFICIENCY ADD:

Press rotate One Nestful Wind

Press rotate Small Celestial Center

Press rotate External Palace of Labor

WITH CHRONIC CONDITION ADD:

Press rotate Two Horses

WITH CONSTIPATION ADD:

Press rotate (clear) Large Intestine Meridian

Push Bone of Seven Segments (downward)

DYSENTERY

Description: Inflammation of mucous membrane of intestinal system.

TCM perspective: Seasonal attack of exogenous pathogens; disharmony of stomach/spleen resulting in qi stagnation, blood stasis, and damaged collaterals.

TCM Differentiation

Damp heat: Fever, abdominal pain, nausea, vomiting, dry lips, thirst, intestinal spasms, stool mixed with blood and/or pus, deep-colored urine.

Tongue: Red with a greasy yellow coating.

Pulse: Rapid and superficial or slippery.

IFV: Purplish red.

Damp cold: White and dilute or white and jellylike stool; abdominal pain; borborygmus; clear, long-passing urine.

Tongue: Red with a greasy white coating.

Pulse: Deep and slow.

IFV: Pale.

Protracted: Stool with pus and/or blood or dry, loose stool with mucus; hot palms and soles; listlessness; weariness; emaciation.

Tongue: Little coating.

Pulse: Deep, thready, and feeble.

IFV: Pale.

Base Protocol

Push, then press rotate Spleen Meridian (clear/tonify)

Push, then press rotate Large Intestine Meridian (clear/tonify)

Push Transport Earth to Water

Rotate push Inner Eight Symbols

Push apart Large Transverse Line

Push Wood Gate

Push Six Hollow Bowels

Grasp Abdominal Corner

Rotate push Abdomen

Press rotate Two Horses

Variations

With damp heat ADD:

Push (clear) Small Intestine Meridian

Push Celestial Gate to Tiger's Mouth

Push Bone of Seven Segments (downward)

Red Phoenix Nods Head

WITH RED STOOL ADD:

Push Water of Galaxy

WITH WHITE STOOL ADD:

Increased repetitions of press rotate Spleen Meridian

WITH DAMP COLD ADD:

Press rotate External Palace of Labor

Press rotate One Nestful Wind

Push Three Passes

Push Bone of Seven Segments (upward)

Medium: Chinese ilex or safflower oil

WITH PROTRACTED CONDITION ADD:

Push Three Passes

Push Bone of Seven Segments (upward)

Medium: Sesame oil or egg white

EARACHE

Description: Pain originating in ear.

TCM perspective: Attack of exogenous wind, cold, or heat pathogens; weak defensive qi; gallbladder/liver inflammation or weakness.

TCM DIFFERENTIATION

Cold: Aversion to cold, headache, no perspiration, dilute nasal discharge.

Tongue: Pale red.

Pulse: Superficial.

IFV: Superficial and light red.

BASE PROTOCOL

Push (clear) Gallbladder Meridian

Press rotate Two Leaf Doors

Press rotate Ear Wind Gate

Push Six Hollow Bowels

Push Bone of Celestial Pillar

Press rotate Auditory Palace

Grasp Wind Pond

Push Water Palace

Push Celestial Gate

Press rotate Great Yang (lightly)

VARIATIONS

WITH FEVER ADD:

Press rotate Inner Palace of Labor

Push Water of Galaxy

WITH COLD ADD:

Press rotate Small Celestial Center

Rotate push Inner Eight Symbols

Press rotate Welcome Fragrance

WITH POOR DIGESTION AND/OR DIARRHEA ADD:

Press rotate Spleen Meridian

Push Below Ribs

Rotate push Abdomen

Press rotate Bubbling Spring

Press rotate Ravine Divide

Press rotate Leg Three Miles

EDEMA

Description: Local or generalized condition in which the body contains excessive amounts of tissue fluid.

TCM perspective: Kidney, lung, and spleen disharmonies; exogenous pathogens.

TCM DIFFERENTIATION

Wind: Causes puffy eyelids initially then spreads all over body, prior to onset: fever, aversion to cold, cough, sore throat, dysuria.

Tongue: Thin white coating.

Pulse: Superficial and rapid.

IFV: Superficial and red.

Damp heat: Oliguria with deep-colored urine, dry stool, vexation, fever, thirst, edema.

Tongue: Red with a yellow coating.

Pulse: Soft, floating, and rapid.

IFV: Bright red or purple.

Kidney/spleen deficiency: Slow onset; facial edema in morning, lower-limb edema in afternoon; sallow complexion; listlessness; weariness; abdominal distension; poor appetite; lumbar aching; cold limbs; oliguria; loose stool.

Tongue: Greasy and white.

Pulse: Deep and slow.

IFV: Pale and deep.

BASE PROTOCOL

Push Liver Meridian back and forth

Push (clear) Small Intestine Meridian

Press rotate Three Yin Meeting

VARIATIONS

WITH WIND ADD:

Push (clear) Lung Meridian

Push (clear) Spleen Meridian

Push (clear) Stomach Meridian

Push Celestial Gate to Tiger's Mouth

Medium: Ginger or scallion decoction

WITH DAMP HEAT ADD:

Push (clear) Lung Meridian

Push (clear) Spleen Meridian

Push (clear) Stomach Meridian

Push Six Hollow Bowels

WITH KIDNEY/SPLEEN YANG DEFICIENCY ADD:

Press rotate Spleen Meridian

Press rotate Kidney Meridian

Press rotate External Palace of Labor

Press rotate Two Horses

Push Three Passes

Medium: Ginger or scallion decoction

ENURESIS

Description: Involuntary discharge of urine after the age when bladder control is expected (approximately five years old).

TCM perspective: Kidney/bladder qi deficiency, spleen/lung qi deficiency, damp heat accumulation in liver meridian.

TCM DIFFERENTIATION

Weak constitution: General deficiency pattern, low energy, weak digestion, low weight, slow growth, pale complexion, child easily contracts colds.

Tongue: Pale.

Pulse: Weak and slow.

IFV: Pale.

Spleen/lung qi deficiency: Emaciation, pale complexion, listlessness, shortness of breath, poor appetite, dripping urine, frequent enuresis with small amounts of urine, loose stool.

Tongue: Pale red with a thin white coating.

Pulse: Slow or deep and thready.

IFV: Pale.

Liver damp heat: Irritability, night sweats, urgent and frequent urination by day, enuresis at night, yellow and foul urine, red complexion and lips.

Tongue: Thin yellow coating.

Pulse: Stringy and slippery.

IFV: Purple.

BASE PROTOCOL

Press rotate Spleen Meridian

Press rotate Kidney Meridian

Push Three Passes

Press rotate External Palace of Labor

Press rotate Elixir Field and Curved Bone, in alternation with rotate push (palm edge) Elixir Field

Press rotate Kidney Back Point

Push Bone of Seven Segments (upward)

Press rotate Three Yin Meeting

Press rotate Meeting of Hundreds

VARIATIONS

WITH WEAK CONSTITUTION AND DEFICIENT OR DEPLETED LOWER BURNER ADD:

Press rotate along both sides of Spinal Column (downward)

Press rotate Two Horses

Press rotate Life Gate

Chafe Life Gate and Eight Sacral Holes

Rub palms together, then cover Life Gate

Medium: Ilex oil or dilute ginger decoction

WITH SPLEEN/LUNG QI DEFICIENCY ADD:

Press rotate Lung Meridian

Press rotate Spleen Back Point

Press rotate Stomach Back Point

Press rotate Heart Back Point

Press rotate Lung Back Point

Medium: Millet decoction

WITH LIVER DAMP HEAT DELETE:

Press rotate Kidney Meridian

Press rotate Kidney Back Point

Press rotate Meeting of Hundreds

AND ADD:

Push (clear) Liver Meridian

Push (clear) Water of Galaxy

Push Transport Earth to Water

Push (clear) Large Intestine Meridian

EPILEPSY

Description: Recurrent spasmodic disorder of the brain with sudden, brief attacks of altered consciousness; motor or sense activity; and recurrent seizure patterns, including possible convulsions.

TCM perspective: Harassed qi due to fright, phlegm obstruction of apertures, heart obstruction by blood stasis.

TCM Differentiation

Blood stasis: Dizziness before onset, quivering lips, chest oppression, palpitations, blurred vision, numb limbs, loss of consciousness, falling, twitching.

Tongue: Purple or red with purplish dots.

Pulse: Slow and uneven.

IFV: Cyanotic.

Phlegm: Faintness, sudden dull appearance, excessive phlegm and slobbering.

Tongue: Thick coating.

Pulse: Stringy and slippery.

IFV: Stagnant and purple.

Base Protocol

Push Liver Meridian back and forth

Fingernail press Small Transverse Lines

Fingernail press, and press rotate Five Digital Joints

Pound Small Celestial Center

Variations

With fever ADD:

Push Six Hollow Bowels

With blood stasis ADD:

Push Water of Galaxy

With phlegm DELETE:

Fingernail press, and press rotate Five Digital Joints

AND ADD:

Push, then press rotate Spleen Meridian (clear, then tonify)

Push Inner Eight Symbols

Push Six Hollow Bowels

EYES, CROSSED

Description: Deviation of one eye toward the other when looking at an object.

TCM perspective: Congenital deficiency, liver disharmony, external pathogenic attack.

BASE PROTOCOL

Press rotate the following bilateral points: Fish Back, Chief Tendon, Four Whites, Tear Container, and Bright Eyes

Push Water Palace and push in a circle around eye orbit

Press rotate Bridge Arch

Grasp Shoulder Well

Press rotate any painful point around eye orbit

EYES, RED OR PAINFUL

Description: Inflammation and dryness around eyes.

TCM perspective: Attack of external wind heat pathogens, liver qi imbalance, yin deficiency or yang excess.

BASE PROTOCOL

Press rotate Blue Tendon

Push Liver Meridian

Press rotate Kidney Line

Press rotate Two Horses

Press rotate Fish Border

Push Water of Galaxy

Push Six Hollow Bowels

Press rotate Bubbling Spring

Grasp Wind Pond

Press rotate Great Yang (lightly)

Push Water Palace

FEVER

Description: Elevation of body temperature above normal.

TCM perspective: Fever results in the struggle between vital qi and pathogenic factors.

TCM DIFFERENTIATION

There are many causes of fever. Listed below are those involving exogenous pathogens.

Wind cold: Cold aversion, no perspiration, clear nasal discharge, headache, itchy throat.

Tongue: Thin white coating.

Pulse: Superficial.

IFV: Superficial and red.

Wind heat: High fever, perspiration, headache, thick nasal discharge, swollen red throat, dry mouth, thirst.

Tongue: Red with a thin yellow or thin white coating.

Pulse: Superficial and rapid.

IFV: Superficial and red-purple.

Lung heat: Cough, fever, aversion to cold, sore throat, stuffy or runny nose with yellow mucus, headache, body aches, slight sweating, thirst, swollen tonsils.

Tongue: Red with a thin white or yellow coating.

Pulse: Floating and rapid.

IFV: Dark purple.

Stomach/spleen deficiency: Sallow complexion, sleepiness, feebleness, poor appetite, abdominal distension, loose stool, restlessness at night, pale lips.

Tongue: Thick, greasy white coating.

Pulse: Thready and weak or slippery.

IFV: Pale and cyanotic.

Summer heat: Aversion to heat, sweating, headache, scanty dark urine, dry lips, thirst.

Tongue: Red.

Pulse: Rapid.

IFV: Deep red and superficial.

Kidney deficiency: Listlessness, reddened eyes, feverish at soles of feet, aversion to clothes, dizziness, limb weakness.

Tongue: Red with a thin coating.

Pulse: Thready and rapid.

IFV: Pale and deep.

BASE PROTOCOL

Fingernail press Old Dragon

Rotate push Inner Palace of Labor

Push Six Hollow Bowels

Press rotate Wind Pond

Push Spinal Column (downward)

Push Celestial Gate

Push Water Palace

Press rotate Great Yang (lightly)

VARIATIONS

WITH WIND COLD ADD:

Press rotate Two Leaf Doors

Push Three Passes

Press rotate One Nestful Wind

Medium: Ginger juice

WITH WIND HEAT ADD:

Push (clear) Lung Meridian

Push, then press rotate Five Digital Joints

Push Water of Galaxy

Medium: Peppermint decoction

WITH LUNG HEAT ADD:

Push (clear) Lung Meridian

Push (clear) Large Intestine Meridian

Push (clear) Stomach Meridian

Press rotate Small Celestial Center

Press rotate One Nestful Wind

Medium: Cool water

WITH STOMACH/SPLEEN DEFICIENCY ADD:

Press rotate Lung Meridian

Push Below Ribs

Rotate push Abdomen

Press rotate Spleen Back Point

Press rotate Bubbling Spring

Press rotate Ravine Divide

Press rotate Leg Three Miles

WITH SUMMER HEAT ADD:

Press rotate Kidney Meridian

Press rotate Small Celestial Center

Press rotate One Nestful Wind

Press Wood Gate

Push Water of Galaxy

Medium: Cool water

WITH KIDNEY DEFICIENCY ADD:

Press rotate Two Horses

Press rotate Inner Palace of Labor

Press rotate Spleen Meridian

Push Water of Galaxy

Press rotate Bubbling Spring

Press rotate Leg Three Miles

FLACCIDITY, FIVE KINDS OF

Description: Relaxed, flabby, poor, or absent muscular tone of neck, mouth, hands, feet, and muscles.

TCM perspective: Congenital deficiency; deficient postnatal nourishment of tendons and muscles.

Tongue: Pale.

Pulse: Thready and feeble.

IFV: Pale and deep.

BASE PROTOCOL

Press rotate Kidney Meridian

Press rotate Two Horses

Rotate push Inner Eight Symbols

Spinal pinch pull (upward)

Push Spinal Column (downward)

Grasp along affected limb

Shake affected limb (gently)

Range of motion affected limb

VARIATIONS

WITH UPPER LIMBS AFFECTED ADD:

Press rotate Pool at the Bend

Press rotate Upper Arm

Press rotate Shoulder Bone

Grasp Union Valley

WITH LOWER LIMBS AFFECTED ADD:

Press rotate Jumping Round

Press rotate Leg Three Miles

Press rotate Suspended Bell

Press rotate Three Yin Meeting

Grasp Ghost Eye

Press rotate Sea of Blood

FURUNCLES

Description: Acute, deep inflammation in skin, usually with suppuration and necrosis; also called boils.

TCM perspective: Qi stagnation or blood stasis caused by exogenous or endogenous heat.

TCM DIFFERENTIATION

Exogenous heat, damp, or wind: Local redness, swelling, and pain; low fever; fretfulness; crying; no desire to eat.

Tongue: Red tip with a thin yellow coating.

Pulse: Superficial and rapid.

IFV: Superficial and bright red.

Endogenous heat: Gradual swelling and enlargement of furuncle, purulent core, severe pain with fever, thirst, constipation.

Tongue: Red with a yellow coating.

Pulse: Superficial and rapid.

IFV: Deep red.

BASE PROTOCOL

Press rotate Small Celestial Center

Press rotate Kidney Meridian

Push Wood Gate

Push apart Large Transverse Line

Push Six Hollow Bowels

VARIATIONS

WITH EXOGENOUS HEAT, DAMP, OR WIND ADD:

Push (clear) Lung Meridian

Press rotate Small Transverse Lines

Rotate push Inner Eight Symbols

Medium: Scute decoction

WITH ENDOGENOUS HEAT ADD:

Increased repetitions of press rotate Small Celestial Center

Press rotate Spleen Meridian

Press rotate Kidney Line

Push Water of Galaxy

GENERAL HEALTH CARE

Description: Preventive care for a generally healthy child to maintain good health and strengthen the constitution.

TCM DIFFERENTIATION

The choice of points and techniques for this protocol is dependent on an accurate general health and constitutional assessment of the child. Signs and patterns may be more difficult to observe when the child is in good health. A good assessment will recognize the underlying patterns and seek to strengthen weaknesses.

BASE PROTOCOL

Press rotate Spleen Meridian

Rotate push Inner Eight Symbols

Push Three Passes

Rotate push Abdomen

Spinal pinch pull (upward)

Press rotate Leg Three Miles

Press rotate Great Yang (lightly)

Press rotate Bubbling Spring

Press rotate Ravine Divide

Push Water Palace

HEADACHE

Description: Different qualities of pain in various regions of the head, acute or chronic.

TCM perspective: There are different patterns involving headache. Only exogenous pathogenic causes are considered here.

TCM DIFFERENTIATION

Wind cold: Ache in neck and back, aversion to wind and cold, dilute nasal discharge, no thirst.

Tongue: Pale red with a thin white coating.

Pulse: Superficial and tense.

IFV: Bright red.

Wind heat: Distended pain in head, aversion to wind and heat, flushing face, conjunctivitis, thirst, desire for drinks, turbid nasal discharge, dry stool, yellow urine.

Tongue: Red with a yellow coating.

Pulse: Superficial and rapid.

IFV: Purplish.

Phlegm turbidity: Eye distension, drooping eyelids, desire to keep eyes closed, nausea, vomiting of sputum and saliva, oppression in chest and epigastric region.

Tongue: Red with a greasy yellow coating.

Pulse: Slippery and rapid.

IFV: Stagnant and purple.

BASE PROTOCOL

Press rotate Two Leaf Doors

Press rotate Union Valley

Press rotate Brain Hollow

Grasp Wind Pond

Push Celestial Gate

Push Water Palace

Press rotate Great Yang (lightly)

VARIATIONS

WITH WIND COLD ADD:

Press rotate One Nestful Wind

Press rotate Small Celestial Center

Press Bamboo Gathering

Medium: Ginger or scallion decoction

WITH WIND HEAT ADD:

Push (clear) Lung Meridian

Press rotate Kidney Line

Push Water of Galaxy

Medium: Peppermint decoction

WITH PHLEGM TURBIDITY ADD:

Press rotate External Palace of Labor

Press rotate Spleen Meridian

Push, then press rotate Small Transverse Lines

HEPATITIS, INFECTIOUS

Description: Infection of the liver.

TCM perspective: Yang jaundice, liver qi stagnation.

TCM DIFFERENTIATION

Heat: Fever, scanty dark-colored urine, fullness and pain of chest/abdomen, jaundice, bitter taste, nausea, vomiting, poor appetite.

Tongue: Red with a sticky yellow coating.

Pulse: Slippery, wiry, and rapid.

IFV: Bright red or purple.

Weak constitution: General deficiency pattern, low energy, weak digestion, low weight, slow growth, pale complexion; child easily contracts colds.

Tongue: Pale.

Pulse: Weak and slow.

IFV: Pale purple.

BASE PROTOCOL

Push Liver Meridian

Push Lung Meridian

Push Stomach Meridian

Push Water of Galaxy

VARIATIONS

WITH HEAT ADD:

Press rotate Small Celestial Center

Press rotate Inner Palace of Labor

Push Six Hollow Bowels

Push Fish for Moon Under Water

WITH DIARRHEA AND WEAK CONSTITUTION ADD:

Press rotate Two Horses

Push, then press rotate Spleen Meridian

Push, then press rotate Kidney Meridian

WITH APPETITE LOSS OR INDIGESTION ADD:

Push Wood Gate

Push Five Digital Joints

Push Six Hollow Bowels

WITH CONSTIPATION ADD:

Push Spleen Meridian

Push Kidney Meridian

Push Bone of Seven Segments (downward)

HERNIA

Description: Protrusion or projection of part of an organ or muscle through the wall of the cavity that normally contains it.

TCM perspective: Exogenous attack of cold, damp, or heat; qi disharmony or deficiency. Clinically: Cold elicits pain, heat elicits relaxation, damp elicits swelling and sinking, deficiency elicits swelling and sinking. A fixed hernia is due to blood disorder, a movable hernia to qi disorder.

TCM DIFFERENTIATION

Damp: Swelling, pain, and dampness of scrotum.

Tongue: White greasy coating.

Pulse: Deep and slow, or deep and tense, or soft, floating, and weak.

IFV: Stagnant and purple.

Cold: Aversion to cold.

Tongue: Pale with little or a white coating.

Pulse: Slow.

IFV: Pale red.

Heat: Aversion to heat.

Tongue: Greasy yellow coating.

Pulse: Soft, floating, and rapid.

IFV: Bright red.

Qi deficiency: Hernial sac bigger when standing, smaller when lying down.

Tongue: Pale.

Pulse: Thready and weak.

IFV: Pale.

Qi depression: Sallow complexion, emaciation, weariness, feebleness, spontaneous perspiration.

Tongue: Pale red with a thin white coating.

Pulse: Slow and feeble.

IFV: Pale and indistinct.

BASE PROTOCOL

Press rotate Two Horses

VARIATIONS

WITH DAMP ADD:

Push, and press rotate Spleen Meridian

Push (clear) Small Intestine Meridian

Push Three Passes

WITH COLD ADD:

Press rotate External Palace of Labor

Press rotate Two Leaf Doors

Press rotate One Nestful Wind

Push Three Passes

WITH HEAT ADD:

Press rotate Small Celestial Center

Press rotate Kidney Line

Push Water of Galaxy

WITH QI DEFICIENCY ADD:

Push, and press rotate Spleen Meridian

Push Three Passes

WITH QI DEPRESSION ADD:

Push Liver Meridian back and forth

Rotate push Inner Eight Symbols

HIVES

Description: Skin reaction or rash characterized by the eruption of pale evanescent wheals with severe itching.

TCM perspective: Attack of exogenous wind, cold, heat, or damp with weak defensive qi or intestinal disruption.

TCM DIFFERENTIATION

Wind heat: Bright red wheals, scorching heat of skin, itching, restlessness, aversion to heat, fretfulness, even swelling of face and lips, symptoms worsen in hot environment and improve in cold.

Tongue: Red with a thin yellow coating.

Pulse: Rapid.

IFV: Red and superficial.

Wind cold: White wheals, serious itching, aversion to cold, fever, symptoms worsen in cold environment.

Tongue: Pale with a white coating.

Pulse: Superficial and tense.

IFV: Pale and superficial.

Wind damp: Pale red wheals, extraordinary itching, symptoms improve in warm environment and worsen on overcast or rainy days.

Tongue: Greasy white coating.

Pulse: Superficial and slippery.

IFV: Red and superficial.

BASE PROTOCOL

Press, then press rotate Small Celestial Center

Press, then press rotate One Nestful Wind

Push apart Large Transverse Line

Push Water of Galaxy

Press, then press rotate Shoulder Well

Press, then press rotate Wind Pond

VARIATIONS

WITH WIND HEAT ADD:

Press rotate External Palace of Labor

Push Six Hollow Bowels

Press rotate Central Islet

Medium: Camphorwood decoction

WITH WIND COLD DELETE:

Push Water of Galaxy

AND ADD:

Press rotate Two Horses

Press rotate Two Leaf Doors

Push Three Passes

Press rotate Great Yang

WITH WIND DAMP ADD:

Push, then press rotate Spleen Meridian

Push Small Intestine Meridian

Fingernail press Union Valley

With recurrent eruptions DELETE:

Push Water of Galaxy

AND ADD:

Press rotate Kidney Meridian

Press rotate Spleen Meridian

Press rotate External Palace of Labor

Press rotate Two Horses

Push Three Passes

Press rotate Leg Three Miles

Medium: Ginger juice

ILEUS

Description: Intestinal obstruction.

TCM perspective: Disharmony of stomach/spleen due to various factors.

TCM Differentiation

Qi stagnation or blood stasis: Abdominal distension, vomiting, abdominal pain throughout year, occasional onset of symptoms, abdominal masses.

Tongue: Thin white coating.

Pulse: Stringy and tense.

IFV: Purplish.

Abdominal qi blockage: Fullness and distension of entire abdomen, tympanic sound upon tapping, abdominal pain, resistance to palpation, intestinal blockage, vomiting, chest oppression, shortness of breath.

Tongue: Greasy coating.

Pulse: Slippery.

IFV: Deep and purple.

Base Protocol

Push (clear) Small Intestine Meridian

Push (clear) Large Intestine Meridian

Rotate push Abdomen

Push Below Ribs

Press rotate Celestial Pivot

Grasp Abdominal Corner

Push Bone of Seven Segments (downward)

VARIATIONS

WITH QI STAGNATION OR BLOOD STASIS ADD:

Rotate push Inner Eight Symbols

Press rotate any painful point on abdomen

Press rotate Lesser Sea

Swift-shifting press

WITH WORMS OR FECAL LUMPS ADD:

Fingernail press, then press rotate Union Valley

Press rotate Abdominal Center

Press rotate Spleen Back Point

Press rotate Stomach Back Point

Fingernail press Pool at the Bend

Press rotate Leg Three Miles

WITH ABDOMINAL QI BLOCKAGE ADD:

Push Liver Meridian back and forth

Push apart Abdominal Yin Yang

WITH FOOD STAGNATION ADD:

Push (clear) Lung Meridian

Push (clear) Stomach Meridian

Press Wood Gate

Fingernail press, then press rotate Leg Three Miles

INFECTIOUS FEBRILE SUMMER DISEASES

Description: Acute, seasonal febrile diseases, mostly occurring in summer or early fall.

TCM perspective: Impaired defensive qi and depletion of qi due to excessive perspiration, which leaves the body susceptible to exogenous attack.

TCM DIFFERENTIATION

Damaged defensive and vital qi: High fever, perspiration, red complexion, headache, lethargy with sober mind, nausea, vomiting, fretfulness, restlessness, convulsions, and twitching.

Tongue: Slightly red with a yellow or white coating.

Pulse: Rapid.

IFV: Bright red.

Damaged qi and yin: Protracted low fever, vexation, thirst, listlessness, feeble breath, abundant perspiration, insomnia, fretfulness, restlessness, poor appetite.

Tongue: Red with little coating.

Pulse: Thready and rapid.

IFV: Bright red.

Genuine yin depletion: Low fever, night sweat, red eyes, vexation, emaciation, dull mind.

Tongue: Red with a glossy surface.

Pulse: Thready and rapid.

IFV: Bright red.

BASE PROTOCOL

Press rotate Two Horses

Press rotate Kidney Meridian

Push apart Large Transverse Line

VARIATIONS

WITH DAMAGED DEFENSIVE AND VITAL QI ADD:

Fingernail press Inner Palace of Labor

Push Water of Galaxy

Push Six Hollow Bowels

Pinch squeeze Celestial Chimney

Pinch squeeze Great Hammer

Grasp Bend Middle

Push Spinal Column (downward)

Medium: Dilute ginger juice

WITH DAMAGED QI AND YIN ADD:

Press rotate Spleen Meridian

Press rotate Small Celestial Center

Press rotate Kidney Summit

Push Three Passes

WITH GENUINE YIN DEPLETION ADD:

Press rotate Small Celestial Center

Push (clear) Lung Meridian

Push (clear) Wood Gate

FOR AFTEREFFECTS ADD:

Press rotate Mute's Gate

Press rotate Jawbone

Grasp Union Valley

Range of Motion all four limbs

JAUNDICE

Description: Symptoms characterized by yellowness of the skin, the whites of the eyes, the mucous membranes, and the body fluids.

TCM perspective: *Yang jaundice:* Accumulated damp heat from exogenous pathogens and spleen damage. *Yin jaundice:* Accumulated damp cold, deficient original qi, and deficient spleen qi.

TCM DIFFERENTIATION

Yang jaundice: Bright yellow skin and sclera, normal mental state, no desire to eat, abdominal distension, constipation, vexation, thirst, nausea, vomiting, oliguria with deep-colored urine.

Tongue: Red with a greasy yellow coating.

Pulse: Slippery and rapid.

IFV: Purplish red.

Yin jaundice: Dim yellow skin and sclera, listlessness, weariness, aversion to cold, oppression in epigastrium, poor appetite, light yellow urine, loose stool.

Tongue: Pale with a greasy white coating.

Pulse: Thready and slow.

IFV: Pale red.

BASE PROTOCOL

Push Liver Meridian back and forth

Press rotate Spleen Meridian

Press rotate Small Celestial Center

Press rotate Kidney Meridian

Push apart Large Transverse Line

Rotate push Inner Eight Symbols (counterflow)

Rotate push Abdomen

VARIATIONS

WITH YANG JAUNDICE ADD:

Push (clear) Lung Meridian

Push Six Hollow Bowels

Push Transport Water to Earth

Fingernail press, then press rotate Four Transverse Lines

Medium: Scallion or musk decoction

WITH YIN JAUNDICE ADD:

Press rotate External Palace of Labor

Press rotate Two Horses

Push, then press rotate Small Transverse Lines

Push Three Passes

Medium: Scallion decoction

LIP DRYNESS AND CREVICES

Description: Dry, cracked, red, painful areas around lips and mouth.

TCM perspective: Arid climate, deficient body fluids, wind heat pathogens attacking the stomach/lage intestine meridians.

BASE PROTOCOL

Push Wood Gate

Push (clear) Spleen Meridian

Press rotate Small Celestial Center

Press rotate Kidney Meridian

Fingernail press, then press rotate Small Transverse Lines

Push Water of Galaxy

Medium: Egg white

MALNUTRITION

Description: Lack of necessary or proper food, or insufficient food absorption or distribution in the body. (This does not include food shortages that cannot be addressed by massage alone. In conditions of poor food availability, malnutrition can continue even after access to food is restored, caused by the following patterns.)

TCM perspective: Primarily damage to the stomach or spleen due to improper feeding patterns or foods, deficiency of blood and qi, or liver stagnation.

TCM Differentiation

Spleen damage by food stasis: Emaciation, sallow complexion, sparse hair, listlessness, tendency to lie down, abdominal distension, vomiting after eating, restless sleep, loose stools or constipation, yellow and turbid urine.

Tongue: Dirty and greasy coating.

Pulse: Slippery and full.

IFV: Pale, purple, and stagnant.

Spleen deficiency: Withered hair, listlessness, weariness, sallow complexion, abdominal distension.

Tongue: Red with a greasy coating.

Pulse: Soft, floating, and slippery.

IFV: Pale purple.

Qi and blood deficiency: Listlessness, slowed development, pale complexion, large head with small neck, sunken abdomen, dry skin, cold limbs, feeble crying, aversion to food, loose stool.

Tongue: Dark red or purple.

Pulse: Tight, wiry, and rapid.

IFV: Stagnant and purple.

Liver stagnation/heat: Blue and sallow complexion, eye symptoms (discharge, pus, watering, redness), emaciation.

Tongue: Dark red or purple.

Pulse: Tight, wiry, and rapid.

IFV: Stagnant and purple.

Note: You may need to treat complications resulting from malnutrition (such as edema, swollen gums, or mouth ulcers) in addition to the above.

Base Protocol

Press rotate Spleen Meridian

Rotate push Inner Eight Symbols

Push Wood Gate

Push Below Ribs

Rotate push Abdomen

Press rotate Leg Three Miles

Variations

With spleen damage by food stasis ADD:

Push (clear) Stomach Meridian

Fingernail press, then press rotate Five Digital Joints

Press rotate Small Celestial Center

Push Three Passes

Medium: Chinese hawthorn decoction

With spleen deficiency ADD:

Press rotate External Palace of Labor

Press rotate Two Horses

Push Three Passes

Push Transport Water to Earth

With qi and blood deficiency ADD:

Press rotate Kidney Meridian

Press rotate Two Horses

Press rotate External Palace of Labor

Push Three Passes

Press rotate Meetings of Hundreds

Medium: Dilute ginger decoction

With liver stagnation/heat ADD:

Push (clear) Liver Meridian

Push Six Hollow Bowels

MEASLES

Description: Acute infectious disease with fever, malaise, sneezing, congestion, cough, conjunctivitis, maculopapular eruptions over entire body.

TCM perspective: The lung, spleen, and sometimes heart may be affected by the resulting fever and depletion of fluids.

TCM DIFFERENTIATION

Favorable course: Three to four days after onset, an even distribution of distinct red, circular spots appears then subsides.

Unfavorable course: Measles remain hidden and closed. The following patterns may appear in an unfavorable course.

Pathogens trapped in lungs: Protracted high fever, serious cough, dyspnea, flaring nostrils, wheezing due to phlegm, incomplete eruption of measles, fretfulness, restlessness, cyanotic lips, cold limbs.

Tongue: Red or crimson with a thin or thick yellow coating.

Pulse: Rapid and superficial or full.

IFV: cyanotic and purple.

Heat sinking into pericardium: Protracted high fever, fretfulness, restlessness, vomiting, convulsions, indistinct consciousness or delirium, faint breath, pale complexion, cold limbs.

Tongue: Red or crimson with a dry yellow coating.

Pulse: Rapid and slippery or full.

IFV: Dim and cyanotic.

Pathogens attacking throat: Throat swelling, pain, hoarseness, irritated cough, vomiting, fretfulness, restlessness, feeling of suffocation.

Tongue: Red with a yellow coating.

Pulse: Superficial and rapid.

IFV: Purple.

BASE PROTOCOL: FAVORABLE COURSE

Push (clear) Lung Meridian

Press rotate Kidney Meridian

Push Three Passes

Press rotate Lung Back Point

Press rotate Spleen Back Point

Press rotate Stomach Back Point

Push Water Palace

Push Celestial Gate

Press rotate Great Yang (lightly)

VARIATIONS

WITH PREMONITORY STAGE ADD:

Push Liver Meridian back and forth

Press rotate Small Celestial Center

Press rotate One Nestful Wind

Push Water of Galaxy

Medium: Dilute ginger juice

WITH ERUPTION STAGE ADD:

Press rotate Two Leaf Doors

Press rotate Small Celestial Center

Press rotate One Nestful Wind

Push Fish for Moon Under Water

Medium: Scute decoction

WITH RECOVERY STAGE ADD:

Press rotate Spleen Meridian

Push Below Ribs

Rotate push Abdomen

Press rotate Leg Three Miles

Press rotate Meeting of Hundreds (lightly)

TO PROMOTE ERUPTIONS ADD:

Increased repetitions of push Three Passes

Press rotate Small Celestial Center

Press rotate Spleen Meridian

Press rotate Two Leaf Doors

BASE PROTOCOL: UNFAVORABLE COURSE

Push (clear) Lung Meridian

Push (clear) Stomach Meridian

Press rotate Wood Gate

Push Liver Meridian back and forth

Rotate push Inner Eight Symbols

Push Water of Galaxy

Push Water Palace

Push Celestial Gate

Press rotate Great Yang (lightly)

VARIATIONS: UNFAVORABLE COURSE

WITH PATHOGENS TRAPPED IN LUNGS ADD:

Pinch squeeze Chest Center

Push apart Scapula

Press rotate along both sides of Spinal Column, especially Heart, Spleen, and Stomach Back Points

Medium: Scute decoction

WITH HEAT SINKING INTO PERICARDIUM ADD:

Press rotate Kidney Meridian

Press rotate Human Center

Press rotate Central Hub

Push, then press rotate Five Digital Joints

Press rotate Inner Palace of Labor

Medium: Coptis decoction

WITH PATHOGENS ATTACKING THROAT ADD:

Push Large Intestine Meridian

Press rotate Palmar Small Transverse Line

Press rotate Celestial Chimney

Fingernail press Pool at the Bend

Fingernail press Lesser Metal Sound

Medium: Coptis decoction

Description: Accumulated milk or food stagnant in the digestive system.

TCM perspective: Spleen/stomach deficiency; improper feeding; overeating of raw, cold, and/or fatty foods.

TCM DIFFERENTIATION

Deficiency and cold: Weakness, pale complexion, feebleness, aversion to cold, cold limbs, poor appetite, loose stool, clear and frequent urination.

Tongue: Pale with a white coating.

Pulse: Slow and feeble.

IFV: Pale red.

Heat: Fever, constipation, aversion to heat, fretfulness, thirst, oliguria with deep-colored urine.

Tongue: Red with a yellow coating.

Pulse: Slippery and rapid.

IFV: Bright red.

BASE PROTOCOL

Push, then press rotate Spleen Meridian

Push, then press rotate Stomach Meridian

Push Liver Meridian back and forth

Rotate push Inner Eight Symbols

Fingernail press, then press rotate Four Transverse Lines

Push Wood Gate

Push Below Ribs

Rotate push Abdomen

Press rotate Leg Three Miles

Medium: Chinese hawthorn decoction

VARIATIONS

WITH DEFICIENCY AND COLD ADD:

Press rotate External Palace of Labor

WITH HEAT ADD:

Push Water of Galaxy

MUMPS

Description: Acute, contagious, febrile disease with inflammation of the parotid and salivary glands.

TCM perspective: Exogenous attack of wind heat; accumulated stagnant damp heat of gallbladder meridian.

TCM DIFFERENTIATION

Wind heat: Fever, headache, pain in cheeks, pain with chewing, poor appetite.

Tongue: Red with a thin white or light yellow coating.

Pulse: Superficial and rapid.

IFV: Superficial and red.

Toxic heat: Fever, headache, dry mouth, nausea, vomiting, listlessness, cheek swelling, pain, constipation, deep-colored urine.

Tongue: Red with a yellow coating.

Pulse: Rapid.

IFV: Purple and stagnant.

BASE PROTOCOL

Push (clear) Liver Meridian

Press rotate Small Celestial Center

Press Wood Gate

Push Six Hollow Bowels

Push Water of Galaxy

Press rotate Bubbling Spring

Press rotate Jawbone

Grasp Wind Pond

Push Water Palace

Press rotate Great Yang (lightly)

Push Celestial Gate

VARIATIONS

WITH WIND HEAT ADD:

Push (clear) Lung Meridian

Press rotate Inner Palace of Labor

Press rotate Two Leaf Doors

Medium: Scallion decoction

WITH TOXIC HEAT ADD:

Press rotate Arm Yang Pool

Push apart Large Transverse Line

Push, then press rotate Four Transverse Lines

Medium: Sesame oil or egg white

WITH SWOLLEN TESTICLES ADD (ADJUNCTIVE TO OTHER THERAPIES):

Press rotate Two Horses

Press rotate Kidney Line

NIGHT CRYING

Description: Sudden crying out at night while sleeping.

TCM perspective: Congenital deficiency of spleen/stomach, postnatal malnutrition, heart fire disturbing shen, fright.

TCM Differentiation

Deficiency and cold: Glossy pale complexion, pale lips, timidity, cold limbs and abdomen, constant low and feeble cry, poor appetite, loose stool.

Tongue: Pale with a thin white coating.

Pulse: Deep and thready.

IFV: Pale red.

Heart fire: Restlessness, aversion to light, sharp and loud crying, red complexion and lips, hot body, constipation, deep-colored urine.

Tongue: Red tip and sides with a white coating.

Pulse: Rapid.

IFV: Dark purple.

Fright: Sudden crying, sudden cyanosis, white complexion and lips, child is easily alarmed.

Tongue: Normal.

Pulse: Abrupt and rapid.

IFV: Black.

Base Protocol

Push apart Large Transverse Line

Press rotate Small Celestial Center

Press rotate Small Transverse Lines

Push Celestial Gate

Push Water Palace

Press rotate Great Yang (lightly)

VARIATIONS

WITH DEFICIENCY AND COLD STOMACH/SPLEEN ADD:

Press rotate Spleen Meridian

Push Three Passes

Push Below Ribs

Rotate push Abdomen

Medium: Ginger or scallion decoction

WITH HEART FIRE ADD:

Push Fish for Moon Under Water

Push (clear) Lung Meridian

Push Water of Galaxy

Medium: Scute decoction or peanut oil

WITH FRIGHT ADD:

Press rotate Heart Meridian

Rotate push Inner Eight Symbols

Red Phoenix Wags Tail

Medium: Peanut oil

PARALYSIS

Description: Temporary suspension or permanent loss of function, especially loss of sensation or motor skills.

TCM perspective: Organs attacked by damp heat, which impacts tendons and meridians; liver/kidney damage; qi and blood deficiency.

TCM DIFFERENTIATION

Lung/stomach pathogens: Fever, nausea, vomiting, body aches, weariness, feebleness, muscle spasms, wheezing due to phlegm in throat, impeded respiration, drowsiness, fretfulness.

Tongue: Greasy white coating.

Pulse: Slippery and rapid.

IFV: Pale.

Damp heat in collaterals: Fever, dry mouth, thirst, stiff neck, twitching, difficult swallowing, deviation of mouth and eyes, constipation, dysuria with deep-colored urine, desires cold drinks.

Tongue: Red with a yellow coating.

Pulse: Slippery and rapid.

IFV: Purple and stagnant.

Liver/kidney depletion: Protracted paralysis, muscular atrophy, limb deformity, inability to coordinate movement.

Tongue: Pale with no coating.

Pulse: Weak and deep.

IFV: Pale and indistinct.

BASE PROTOCOL

Push Liver Meridian back and forth

Push (clear) Lung Meridian

Push apart Large Transverse Line

Press rotate Small Celestial Center

Push Water of Galaxy

Press rotate Spinal Column, especially Lung, Spleen, and Stomach Back Points

Press Shoulder Well

Press rotate any painful point in affected region

Range of motion affected areas

VARIATIONS

WITH LUNG/STOMACH PATHOGENS ADD:

Press rotate One Nestful Wind

Push Wood Gate

Push (clear) Small Intestine Meridian

Fingernail press Four Transverse Lines

Medium: Peppermint decoction

WITH DAMP HEAT IN COLLATERALS ADD:

Fingernail press Jawbone

Fingernail press Earth Granary

Grasp Ghost Eye

Grasp Front Mountain Support

Grasp Bend Middle

Rotate push Three Yin Meeting

WITH LIVER/KIDNEY DEPLETION DELETE:

Push Liver Meridian

Push Lung Meridian

Push apart Large Transverse Line

Push Water of Galaxy

AND ADD:

Press rotate Spleen Meridian

Press rotate Kidney Meridian

Press rotate Lung Meridian

Press rotate Two Horses

Press rotate Meeting of Hundreds

Push Three Passes

Push Wood Gate to Large Transverse Line

PERSPIRATION

Description: Secretion of salty fluid through the sweat glands of the skin.

TCM perspective: Exterior deficiency, yang deficiency heat due to accumulated stasis, deficiency fire due to deficient yin.

TCM DIFFERENTIATION

Exterior deficiency: Aversion to wind and cold; spontaneous perspiration, especially with activity; feebleness; headache; chills; listlessness.

Tongue: Pale with a white coating.

Pulse: Thready and weak.

IFV: Pale.

Yang deficiency: Cold-feeling body; aversion to cold; no perspiration of hands or feet; pale complexion; weakness; frequent perspiration, especially with activity; poor appetite; loose stool; dysuria; yellow urine.

Tongue: Pale with a greasy yellow coating.

Pulse: Soft, floating, and rapid.

IFV: Pale and deep.

Excess heat: High fever, thirst, continuous perspiration, abdominal distension, poor appetite, irregular bowel movements.

Tongue: Dry and yellow coating.

Pulse: Full and rapid.

IFV: Deep purple.

Deficiency fire: Night sweats, emaciation, fretfulness, red eyes, afternoon fever, heart palpitations, restlessness, dry stool, yellow urine.

Tongue: Red with little coating.

Pulse: Thready and rapid.

IFV: Pale purple.

BASE PROTOCOL

Press rotate Two Horses

Press rotate Kidney Meridian

Press rotate Kidney Summit

Push Wood Gate

Press rotate Small Celestial Center

VARIATIONS

WITH EXTERIOR DEFICIENCY ADD:

Press rotate One Nestful Wind

Push apart Large Transverse Line

Push Water of Galaxy

WITH YANG DEFICIENCY ADD:

Press rotate Lung Meridian

Spinal pinch pull

Press rotate Spleen Back Point

Press rotate Stomach Back Point

Press rotate Kidney Back Point

Push Three Passes

WITH EXCESS HEAT ADD:

Press rotate One Nestful Wind

Push, then press rotate Small Transverse Lines

Push Water of Galaxy

Push Six Hollow Bowels

WITH DEFICIENCY FIRE ADD:

Press rotate External Palace of Labor

Push apart Large Transverse Line

Rotate push Inner Eight Symbols

Push Fish for Moon Under Water

PHLEGM CONDITIONS, CHRONIC

Description: Recurrent episodes of thick mucus.

TCM perspective: Improper transformation of fluids impairing spleen function, weak defensive qi with attack of exogenous pathogens, poor diet leading to spleen-deficiency patterns.

BASE PROTOCOL

Press rotate Spleen Meridian

Rotate push Inner Eight Symbols

Push, then press rotate Five Digital Joints

Press rotate Wood Gate

Push Three Passes

Push Below Ribs

Rotate push Abdomen

Spinal pinch pull, especially Spleen Back Point

Press rotate Bubbling Spring

Press rotate Ravine Divide

Press rotate Leg Three Miles

VARIATIONS

WITH HEAD CONGESTION ADD:

Press rotate External Place of Labor

Press rotate Welcome Fragrance

Grasp Wind Pond

Push Celestial Gate

Push Water Palace

Press rotate Great Yang

WITH LUNG CONGESTION ADD:

Press rotate Lung Meridian

Push apart Chest Center

Press rotate Lung Back Point

WITH EARACHE ADD:

Press rotate Two Leaf Doors

Press rotate Ear Wind Gate

PNEUMONIA

Description: Lung inflammation caused by a variety of factors.

TCM perspective: Wind heat external pathogen attack of lung, with possible kidney involvement.

BASE PROTOCOL

Press rotate One Nestful Wind

Rotate push (counterflow) Inner Eight Symbols (clears Lung and Liver Meridians)

Press rotate Palmar Small Transverse Line

Push Small Transverse Lines

Push Wood Gate

Push Water of Galaxy

Press rotate Lung Back Point

VARIATIONS

WITH PERSISTENT FEVER ADD:

Pinch squeeze along both sides of Celestial Chimney to xiphoid process

Pinch squeeze Great Hammer

Pinch squeeze Central Treasury

Pound Fish Border

Rotate push Inner Palace of Labor

Press rotate Yang Marsh

Press rotate Great Yang

Push Water Palace

Push Celestial Gate

Grasp Wind Pond

PROLAPSED RECTUM

Description: Protrusion of rectal mucosa through the anus.

TCM perspective: Stagnant heat in the middle and/or lower burner; fragile qi, especially spleen and kidney.

TCM Differentiation

Stagnant heat in middle or lower burner: Constipation; hot abdomen at night; hot, red, swollen, painful anus.

Tongue: Red with a thin yellow coating.

Pulse: Rapid.

IFV: Purple or deep red.

Fragile qi: Sallow complexion, emaciation, weariness, feebleness, spontaneous perspiration, red prolapsed rectum with no pain.

Tongue: Pale with a thin white coating.

Pulse: Slow and feeble.

IFV: Pale.

Base Protocol: Stagnant Heat in Middle or Lower Burner

Press rotate Spleen Meridian

Push (clear) Large Intestine Meridian

Push Water of Galaxy

Push Below Ribs

Rotate push Abdomen

Push Bone of Seven Segments (downward)

Press rotate Meeting of Hundreds

VARIATIONS

WITH CONSTIPATION ADD:

Press rotate Small Celestial Center

Press rotate Wood Gate

Push Six Hollow Bowels

BASE PROTOCOL: FRAGILE QI

Press rotate Lung Meridian

Press rotate Kidney Meridian

Press rotate External Palace of Labor

Press rotate Spleen Back Point

Push Bone of Seven Segments (upward)

Press rotate Tortoise Tail

Press rotate Meeting of Hundreds

VARIATIONS

WITH INCREASED WEAKNESS ADD:

Press rotate Two Horses

Spinal pinch pull

RETARDATION, FIVE KINDS OF

Description: Delayed development of standing, walking, teething, speaking, and hair growth.

TCM perspective: Congenital deficiency, deficient postnatal nutrition, deficient qi and blood.

TCM DIFFERENTIATION

Kidney/liver deficiency: Weakness, atrophy of limbs, inability to stand or walk, retardation of teething, delayed obliteration of fontanel.

Tongue: Pale red with no coating.

Pulse: Deep and thready.

IFV: Pale purple.

Heart/spleen deficiency: Mental dullness, inability to speak, withered and fragile hair, sallow complexion, pale lips.

Tongue: Pale with a thin coating.

Pulse: Feeble and deficient.

IFV: Pale.

BASE PROTOCOL

Press rotate Two Horses

Press rotate Spleen Meridian

Press rotate Kidney Meridian

Push apart Large Transverse Line

Push Three Passes

VARIATIONS

WITH KIDNEY/LIVER DEFICIENCY ADD:

Push Liver Meridian back and forth

Press rotate External Palace of Labor

WITH HEART/SPLEEN DEFICIENCY ADD:

Press rotate Small Celestial Center

Rotate push Inner Eight Symbols

Fingernail press Four Transverse Lines

Press rotate Yang Marsh

RICKETS

Description: Abnormal shape and structure of bones in developing children due to inadequate formation of cartilage.

TCM perspective: Deficiency and weakness of spleen and kidney.

TCM DIFFERENTIATION

Stomach/spleen deficiency: Puffy face, lazy talking, mental dullness, weakness, hyperhidrosis, vexation, insomnia, flaccid muscles, soft skull, wide and retarded obliteration of the fontanel, sparse and sallow hair, loose stool, child is easily frightened.

Tongue: Thin white coating.

Pulse: Slow and feeble.

IFV: Pale red.

Kidney depletion: Emaciation; pale complexion; retardation of standing, walking, hair growth, teething, and speaking; pigeon breast; tortoise back; obvious deformity of bones; swollen abdomen; crooked legs.

Tongue: Pale with little coating.

Pulse: Slow and feeble.

IFV: Pale.

BASE PROTOCOL

Press rotate Kidney Meridian

Press rotate Spleen Meridian

Push Three Passes

Press rotate Spleen Back Point

Press rotate Stomach Back Point

Rotate push Abdomen

VARIATIONS

WITH STOMACH/SPLEEN DEFICIENCY ADD:

Push Transport Earth to Water

Spinal pinch pull

Press rotate Abdominal Center

Rotate push Eight Sacral Holes

WITH KIDNEY DEPLETION ADD:

Press rotate Lung Meridian

Press rotate Heart Meridian

Press rotate Meeting of Hundreds

Press rotate Lung Back Point

Press rotate Heart Back Point

RUBELLA

Description: Acute infectious disease similar to scarlet fever and measles but differing in its shorter course, slight fever, and lack of aftereffects. Also called German measles.

TCM perspective: Weak exterior defenses allow for attack by seasonal pathogens of wind heat.

BASE PROTOCOL: DURING ERUPTIONS

Press rotate Spleen Meridian

Press rotate Small Celestial Center

Press rotate One Nestful Wind

Push (clear) Lung Meridian

Push Three Passes

Grasp Wind Pond

Grasp Shoulder Well

BASE PROTOCOL: AFTER ERUPTIONS

Press rotate Kidney Meridian

Press rotate Spleen Meridian

Press rotate Kidney Line

Push Wood Gate

Push apart Large Transverse Line

Press rotate Small Celestial Center

Push Water of Galaxy

Medium: Scallion decoction

VARIATIONS*

WITH HIGH FEVER DELETE:

Push Water of Galaxy

AND ADD:

Push Six Hollow Bowels

Push (clear) Lung Meridian

Rotate push Inner Palace of Labor

WITH POOR APPETITE ADD:

Push (clear) Stomach Meridian

Push Below Ribs

Rotate push Abdomen

WITH SORE THROAT ADD:

Pinch squeeze Celestial Chimney

Fingernail press Lesser Metal Sound

---

* Variations may be used either during or after eruptions.

SKIN ERUPTIONS

Description: Acute condition with a high fever; a diffuse maculopapular rash appears when the fever suddenly subsides.

TCM perspective: Seasonal attack of wind, with damp heat in the spleen or lung.

BASE PROTOCOL

Press rotate Kidney Meridian

Push Liver Meridian back and forth

Press rotate Small Celestial Center

Push Wood Gate

Push Water of Galaxy

VARIATIONS

WITH FEVER STAGE ADD:

Press rotate One Nestful Wind

Push apart Large Transverse Line

Push Celestial Gate

Medium: Cold water

WITH ERUPTION STAGE ADD:

Press rotate Spleen Meridian

Press rotate Two Horses

Fingernail press Small Transverse Lines

WITH VOMITING ADD:

Push Stomach Meridian

SORE THROAT

Description: Inflammation of the throat, tonsils, pharynx, or larynx.

TCM perspective: Exogenous wind cold or wind heat pathogen attack.

BASE PROTOCOL

Push (clear) Lung Meridian

Press rotate Union Valley

Rotate push Inner Eight Symbols

Grasp Wind Pond

Press Celestial Chimney

Chafe Bridge Arch

Push Water of Galaxy

Push Celestial Gate

Push Water Palace

Press rotate Great Yang (lightly)

STIFFNESS, FIVE KINDS OF

Description: Stiffness of neck, mouth, hands, feet, and muscles, sometimes seen in premature newborns.

TCM perspective: Congenital deficiency with exogenous wind cold attack causing deficient nourishment of local area, resulting in qi stagnation and blood stasis.

BASE PROTOCOL

Press rotate Spleen Meridian

Press rotate Kidney Meridian

Press rotate Two Horses

Press rotate External Palace of Labor

Rotate push Inner Eight Symbols

Fingernail press Yang Marsh

Fingernail press Yang Mound Spring

Fingernail press Jumping Round

Press, then rub roll stiff body parts

STRABISMUS

Description: Eye disorder in which the eyes cannot both look toward the same object.

TCM perspective: Congenital deficiency, liver disharmony, external pathogenic attack.

BASE PROTOCOL

Press rotate with thumb: any painful point around eye, Fish Back, Pupil Bone Hole, Bright Eyes, Bamboo Gathering, and Tear Container; repeat several times for a total of 15–20 minutes.

Press Great Yang (hold deep)

Press rotate Wind Pond

Grasp Shoulder Well

VARIATIONS

OPTIONAL POINTS:

Press rotate Upper Arm

Fingernail press Symmetric Upright

SWOLLEN GUMS

Description: Local inflammation and swelling in the gums of the mouth.

TCM perspective: Attack of exogenous pathogens with accumulated heat and stagnation in the large intestine and/or stomach meridians.

Tongue: Red with a yellow coating.

Pulse: Rapid.

IFV: Bright red or purple.

BASE PROTOCOL

Push Spleen Meridian

Press rotate Union Valley

Press rotate Kidney Meridian

Push (clear) Small Intestine Meridian

Press rotate Small Celestial Center

Push Six Hollow Bowels

Push Water of Galaxy

Medium: Peanut or paraffin oil

WITH UPPER GUM **ADD:**

Push Wood Gate

WITH LOWER GUM **ADD:**

Push (clear) Large Intestine Meridian

Push (clear) Lung Meridian

TEETHING OR TOOTHACHE

Description: Eruption of teeth through gums; pain in or around tooth.

TCM perspective: Attack of exogenous pathogens, uprising stomach fire, deficient fire due to depletion of kidney yin.

TCM DIFFERENTIATION

Excess: Bad breath, even swelling of gum and cheek, headache, fever, constipation.

Tongue: Yellow coating.

Pulse: Superficial and rapid.

IFV: Superficial and deep red.

Deficiency: Vague toothache, no swelling of gum or cheek.

Tongue: Glossy with no coating.

Pulse: Thready and rapid.

IFV: Pale red.

BASE PROTOCOL

Press rotate Kidney Meridian

Press rotate Small Celestial Center

Press rotate or fingernail press Chief Tendon

Push Water Palace

Press rotate Great Yang

Push Celestial Gate

VARIATIONS

WITH TOOTHACHE AND EXCESS **ADD:**

Press rotate One Nestful Wind

Push Water of Galaxy

Press rotate Broken Sequence

WITH TOOTHACHE AND DEFICIENCY ADD:

Press rotate Two Horses

Press rotate Union Valley

Press rotate Spleen Meridian

PAIN RELIEF POINTS:

Press rotate Union Valley

Push Six Hollow Bowels

Press rotate Leg Three Miles

Press rotate Before Vertex

Press rotate Ear Wind Gate

THRUSH

Description: Infection of the mouth or throat that features white patches and ulcers sometimes accompanied by fever and gastrointestinal inflammation. Also called aphtha, sprue, or stomatitis.

TCM perspective: Excess or deficient yin fire affecting the heart, spleen, or kidney yin.

TCM DIFFERENTIATION

Excess fire: Red complexion and lips, restlessness, white ulcers in mouth and tongue, constipation, deep-colored urine.

Tongue: Red tipped.

Pulse: Rapid and full.

IFV: Purple and stagnant.

Deficient yin fire: Weakness, timidity, pale complexion with red eyes, hot palms and soles, no thirst, low fever, night sweat.

Tongue: Red with little coating.

Pulse: Thready and feeble.

IFV: Pale red.

BASE PROTOCOL

Push (clear) Small Intestine Meridian

Press rotate Chief Tendon

Push Wood Gate

Push, then Press rotate Small Transverse Lines

Press rotate Small Celestial Center

Push Water of Galaxy

VARIATIONS

WITH EXCESS FIRE ADD:

Push (clear) Stomach Meridian

Push (clear) Lung Meridian

Push apart Large Transverse Line

Press rotate Inner Palace of Labor

Push Fish for Moon Under Water

WITH DEFICIENT YIN FIRE ADD:

Press rotate Kidney Meridian

Press rotate Spleen Meridian

Rotate push Inner Eight Symbols

Press rotate Two Horses

Push Below Ribs

Rotate push Abdomen

Spinal pinch pull, especially Spleen and Kidney Back Points

Medium: Scallion decoction

TORTICOLLIS

Description: Stiff neck caused by the spasmodic contraction of neck muscles; the chin or ear may be drawn to one side. Also called wryneck.

TCM perspective: Trauma to sternocleidomastoid muscle during delivery; attack of exogenous wind cold.

BASE PROTOCOL

Press rotate with thumb Bridge Arch, alternating with grasp Bridge Arch

Range of motion: stretch Bridge Arch by lateral movement, then rotate head left and right

VARIATIONS

OPTIONAL POINTS:

Press, or grasp Shoulder Well

ON AFFECTED SIDE:

Fingernail press Broken Sequence

Press rotate Jumping Round (lightly)

Press rotate Three Yin Meeting (lightly)

DAILY HOME EXERCISES:

Stretch Bridge Arch

Range of motion neck

URINATION, FREQUENT

Description: Urination frequency increases to more than normal.

TCM perspective: Kidney yang deficiency.

BASE PROTOCOL

Press rotate Kidney Meridian

Press rotate Two Horses

Press rotate Three Yin Meeting

Press rotate Fish Border

Rotate push Elixir Field

Press rotate Kidney Back Point

URINE RETENTION

Description: Inability to urinate or fully urinate when necessary.

TCM perspective: Congenital deficiency; weak original qi; qi disorder; damp/heat attacking lung, spleen, or kidney.

TCM DIFFERENTIATION

Qi deficiency: Glossy pale complexion, cold limbs, listlessness, clear urine, dripping urine, feeble urine discharge.

Tongue: Pale with a thin coating.

Pulse: Thready and weak.

IFV: Pale red.

Damp heat: Deep-colored and turbid urine, pain, distended lower abdomen, thirst, fretfulness, restlessness.

Tongue: Greasy yellow coating.

Pulse: Slippery and rapid.

IFV: Purple or red.

BASE PROTOCOL

Press rotate Spleen Meridian

Rotate push Inner Eight Symbols

Push (clear) Small Intestine Meridian

Press rotate Two Horses

Push Three Passes

Rotate push (with palm edge) Elixir Field

Push Winnower Gate

VARIATIONS

WITH QI DEFICIENCY ADD:

Press rotate Kidney Meridian

Press rotate External Palace of Labor

Press rotate Leg Three Miles

Medium: Peanut oil

WITH DAMP HEAT DELETE:

Push Three Passes

AND ADD:

Press rotate Small Celestial Center

Push Water of Galaxy

Press rotate Arm Yang Pool

VOMITING

Description: Ejection through mouth of gastric contents.

TCM perspective: Attack of exogenous pathogens, overeating or overdrinking, falling, fright, accumulation of heat or cold in stomach from congenital deficiency or deficient stomach qi.

TCM DIFFERENTIATION

Wind cold: Sudden onset, frequent vomiting, cold aversion, no perspiration.

Tongue: Pale red.

Pulse: Superficial and slow.

IFV: Reddish.

Wind heat: Sudden onset, frequent vomiting, fever and/or chills, perspiration, headache, itchy throat.

Tongue: Red with a thin white or greasy yellow coating.

Pulse: Superficial and rapid.

IFV: Purple.

Abnormal diet: Fullness, pain at epigastric region, foul gas belching, sour and putrid vomiting, fretfulness, insomnia, constipation or diarrhea, symptoms relieved with vomiting.

Tongue: Thick with a greasy coating.

Pulse: Slippery.

IFV: Dim and stagnant.

Stomach heat: Vomiting soon after eating, fretfulness, restlessness, red complexion and lips, constipation, deep-colored urine, desires liquids.

Tongue: Red with a yellow coating.

Pulse: Rapid.

IFV: Red or purple.

Stomach cold: Recurrent vomiting, clear and dilute vomit without foul odor, pale complexion and lips, cold limbs, continuous abdominal pain, loose stool.

Tongue: Pale with a white coating.

Pulse: Deep, thready, and feeble.

IFV: Pale red.

Flaming deficient yin fire: Endogenous fever, dry mouth and throat, poor appetite, hot soles and palms, fever, night sweat, dry stool.

Tongue: Red with little coating.

Pulse: Thready and rapid.

IFV: Pale purple.

BASE PROTOCOL

Fingernail press Maternal Cheek

Rotate push Inner Eight Symbols

Push (clear) Small Intestine Meridian

Push (clear) Stomach Meridian

Press Wood Gate

Push Below Ribs

Rotate push Abdomen

Push Bone of Celestial Pillar (downward)

Press rotate Spleen Back Point

Press rotate Bubbling Spring

Press rotate Ravine Divide

Press rotate Leg Three Miles

Push Water Palace

VARIATIONS

WITH WIND COLD ADD:

Press rotate Two Leaf Doors

Press rotate Lung Back Point

Push Celestial Gate

Medium: Ginger juice or decoction

WITH WIND HEAT ADD:

Press rotate Union Valley

Push Six Hollow Bowels

Press rotate Great Hammer

Medium: Peppermint decoction

WITH ABNORMAL DIET ADD:

Push (clear) Large Intestine Meridian

Increased repetitions of push Below Ribs

Press rotate all points along both sides of Spinal Column, especially Spleen and
    Stomach Back Points

Medium: Ginger juice

WITH STOMACH HEAT ADD:

Push Water of Galaxy

Push Transport Earth to Water

Push Large Transverse Line to Wood Gate

WITH STOMACH COLD ADD:

Press rotate External Palace of Labor

Push Three Passes

Spinal pinch pull, especially Spleen Back Point

Rub palms together, then cover Elixir Field

Medium: Ginger decoction

WITH FLAMING DEFICIENT YIN FIRE ADD:

Press rotate Two Horses

Push Water of Galaxy

Push Spinal Column (downward)

WHOOPING COUGH

Description: Acute infectious disease with recurrent spasms of coughing ending in an inspiration with a characteristic "whoop" sound.

TCM perspective: Weak constitution; seasonal attack of pathogens.

TCM DIFFERENTIATION

Intermediate stage: Recurrent, sudden, irritated coughing; gasping for breath; flushed face to ears; clenched fists; protruding jugular vein; symptoms worsen at night; each series of coughs may be repeated successively until after the last cough the child inhales, making a "whoop" sound; spasms may include vomiting.

Tongue: Red with a thick yellow or white coating.

Pulse: Slippery and rapid.

IFV: Purple and stagnant.

Advanced stage: Feebleness, fewer episodes of coughing, listlessness, weariness, poor appetite, unusual urination and bowel movement habits, spontaneous perspiration, night sweats, unproductive cough, hot palms and soles.

Tongue: Pale with a thin coating.

Pulse: Thready and feeble.

IFV: Dim and pale.

BASE PROTOCOL

Press rotate Spleen Meridian

Push (clear) Lung Meridian

Press rotate Kidney Meridian

Press rotate Small Intestine Meridian

Fingernail press Vim Tranquillity

Press rotate One Nestful Wind

Rotate push Inner Eight Symbols

Push apart Chest Center

Swift-shifting press

Push Water Palace

Press rotate Great Yang (lightly)

VARIATIONS

WITH INTERMEDIATE STAGE ADD:

Push Celestial Gate to Tiger's Mouth

Push Water of Galaxy

Press Celestial Chimney

Push apart Abdominal Yin Yang

WITH ADVANCED STAGE ADD:

Push Three Passes

Press rotate all points along both sides of Spinal Column, especially Lung, Spleen, Stomach, and Kidney Back Points

Red Phoenix Nods Head

DURING SPASMODIC ATTACK ADD:

Press rotate Small Celestial Center

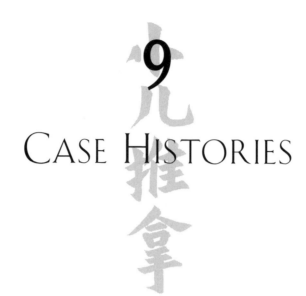

CASE HISTORIES

THIS CHAPTER PRESENTS CASE HISTORIES that demonstrate the clinical application of Chinese pediatric massage. I selected these cases because they exemplify aspects either of pediatric massage or of how CPM applications change with the child.

Of course the treatment plans presented in chapter 8, Protocols, are in essence case histories of treating specific patterns. When a child conforms to the given assessment, application of the appropriate protocols will generally produce good results. But the truth is that children rarely present an easy, classic TCM syndrome. Instead, many factors must go into an overall treatment plan, including the child's energetic condition, the parents, and other treatment modalities. Thus the following cases should help you adapt the protocols to fit your own patients.

ENURESIS

Child information: Six-year-old female, average height and weight.

Presenting symptoms: Bed-wetting at night five out of seven nights.

History: The child had a history of infrequent enuresis, which seemed to have resolved. When she began school, however, symptoms recurred.

Assessment: Shen: eyes and complexion slightly dull, withdrawn; lips: very red, chapped; pulse: slow; abdomen: gurgling sounds.

TCM differentiation: Slight kidney deficiency, affecting heart and bladder.

FIRST CPM TREATMENT

Press rotate Spleen Meridian

Press rotate Kidney Meridian

Press rotate External Palace of Labor

Press rotate Two Horses

Push Three Passes

Rotate push Abdomen

Rotate push (palm edge) Elixir Field

Press rotate Curved Bone

Press rotate Spinal Column, especially Kidney Back Point

Press rotate Life Gate

Chafe, then rub palms together and warm Life Gate

Push Bone of Seven Segments (upward)

Press rotate Bubbling Spring

Press rotate Ravine Divide

Press rotate Leg Three Miles

Push Celestial Gate

Push Water Palace

Press rotate Great Yang

Press rotate Meeting of Hundreds

HOME TREATMENT

Press rotate Spleen and Kidney Meridians

Rotate push Abdomen

TREATMENT RESPONSE

After the first treatment the frequency of enuresis was reduced from five nights per week to two nights per week.

SECOND TREATMENT

The treatment for the second visit was unchanged from the first. The techniques were reinforced by adding the Chinese herbal formula Golden Lock Pill: one pill two times per day.

FOLLOW-UP

Compliance with the herbal pill was good. A follow-up call three months later revealed that the enuresis occurred twice in the weeks following the second treatment and then ceased completely.

This case is an example of a pediatric condition that Western medicine does not address well, but for which pediatric massage has a very high success rate. While seemingly a bit old for pediatric massage, this child's energetic physiology was slightly immature for her age. Thus, she responded well and quickly to the techniques. This child also responded very deeply to the abdominal techniques. Rectifying the center greatly contributed to astringing the kidney essence. Another important aspect in this case was warming the kidney by manipulating Life Gate.

ABDOMINAL PAIN—INFANT

Child information: Two-week-old female, six pounds, nineteen inches.

Presenting symptoms: Abdominal pain, digestive difficulty.

History: Normal delivery. The child curls in a ball as if her stomach hurts, usually once per day for up to three hours. Western medications have been tried with little effect. The mother has chronic irritable bowel syndrome.

Assessment: Abdomen: very tense; tongue: thick white coating; IFV: slight appearance at first gate.

TCM differentiation: Middle-burner weakness.

FIRST CPM TREATMENT

Press rotate Spleen Meridian

Push Small Intestine Meridian

Rotate push Inner Eight Symbols

Push Three Passes

Rotate push Abdomen

Push Below Ribs

Press rotate along both sides of Spinal Column, especially Spleen Back Point

Spinal pinch pull

Press rotate Tortoise Tail

Press rotate Bubbling Spring

Press rotate Ravine Divide

Press rotate Leg Three Miles

Push Celestial Gate

Push Water Palace

Press rotate Great Yang

HOME TREATMENT

Press rotate Spleen Meridian

Rotate push Abdomen

TREATMENT RESPONSE

After the first treatment the parent reported the child was without pain symptoms for five days.

SECOND TREATMENT

Assessment at the second treatment included a slightly flushed face with small red dots, restlessness, and irritability. The tongue was red tipped. In addition to middle-warmer weakness, the child now had a slight heat condition. The treatment was thus changed to include: press rotate Small Celestial Center, push apart Large Transverse Line, and push Water of Galaxy.

FOLLOW-UP

The treatment continued twice each week for four weeks. The severity, frequency, and length of the symptoms decreased gradually until they were gone by the fourth week.

Reflective of the quickly changing nature of infants, this child presented heat signs in the second week, constipation in the third week, and occasional diarrhea throughout. Protocols were adapted according to each change.

In addition, an external herbal remedy was started during the second week of treatment (scallion, ginger, and bran paste). This formula dispelled cold and warmed the middle burner. It was very effective for short-term use, with almost immediate relief of symptoms upon application.

After several weeks without symptoms (or treatment) the mother stopped breast-feeding and began using infant formula. Within several days the child began experiencing abdominal symptoms again, although slightly different from those of the previous month.

The new condition reflected spleen-deficiency cold, probably due to the change from breast milk to formula. The treatment protocol was adapted to focus on warming the spleen and promoting intestinal movement. In addition to the base treatment above, the following points were used: Five Digital Joints; Small Intestine, Large Intestine, and Stomach Meridians; and Six Hollow Bowels.

Different types of formula were tried with varying degrees of tolerance. As the mother experimented with formula, the abdominal pain and constipation were kept relatively minor with twice-weekly treatments for six weeks. Reducing the frequency of treatments resulted in a return of symptoms.

An internal herbal formula (Peony and Licorice Combination) was given in the third week of the second condition, with good results.

After the second series of treatments, the child was without digestive problems until solid foods were introduced. Periodic treatments continued as needed for several months and then were discontinued as unnecessary.

COMMENTS

This case presents a good example of a newborn condition that is simple, yet can cause many difficulties for both parent and child. The treatment is very light, due to the age of the infant—her skin is still easily irritated. In a case like this one to three treatments are usually sufficient to restore balance. However, the complicating factor here is the mother's chronic abdominal condition.

Part of the first session was spent discussing with the mother the ways in which her condition relates to her daughter, and that taking care of herself will help care for the child. This is a good example of treating the mother to treat the child. The first several treatments produced a strong response from the child, which lasted for a number of days afterward. After four weeks the child's middle burner was much stronger and without symptoms.

The second phase of treatment reflects the basic middle-burner weakness relative to adapting to changes, in this case from breast milk to formula (later to solid foods). With regular treatments for another six weeks, the middle burner returned to balance. This condition may be due to an inherited weakness and will be followed with a constitution-strengthening program. The mother is interested in learning about the energetics of foods and will continue home care.

FIVE KINDS OF STIFFNESS/RETARDATION (PERTHES' DISEASE)

Child information: Five-year-old male, low-average weight and height.

Presenting symptoms: Pain, restricted range of motion, tight muscles in right leg/hip. Western medical diagnosis: Perthes' disease, confirmed by X rays. *Perthes' disease* describes irregularities in the formation of bone from cartilage in the head of the femur, with resulting deformed growth patterns.

History: Child complained of leg pain after high-movement activities for several months prior to diagnosis.

Assessment: Good general signs; tongue: slightly pale; right leg, especially lateral aspect: very tense relative to left leg.

TCM differentiation: Slight kidney deficiency; poor bone development causing muscular stiffness.

FIRST CPM TREATMENT

Rub Roll

Knead*

Roll*

One Finger Pushing*

All techniques performed on anterior and posterior right leg, except for local pain area at femoral head.

HOME TREATMENT

Application of bone-nourishing liniment externally one to two times per day.

TREATMENT RESPONSE

The purpose of the first treatment was to assess how the child would tolerate vigorous massage techniques. Both child and parent reported good results from the first treatment. The child felt less tension in his leg and fewer episodes of pain, which came and went.

SECOND TREATMENT

Added to the first treatment techniques were:

Press rotate Spleen Meridian

Press rotate Kidney Meridian

Press rotate Two Horses

Press rotate External Palace of Labor

Rotate push Abdomen

Press rotate all points along both sides of Spinal Column, especially Spleen and Kidney Back Points

Spinal pinch pull

Press rotate Yang Mound Spring

FOLLOW-UP

Treatments were given once per week for three weeks until there was no more pain in the right leg and the differences between right- and left-leg tension were diminished. Six more treatments were given at intervals of two weeks. The child

---

* These are adult tui na techniques and are not described in this book.

was also taking vitamin and mineral supplements.

At the end of this period the orthopedic physician performed a follow-up X ray and found the femoral head to be normal. The physician was pleased and surprised at this rate of progress; the standard duration of this condition is one year or more, yet this case resolved in five months.

COMMENTS

This case shows a combination pattern from five kinds of stiffness and retardation. The retardation was related to the normal development of cartilage into bone at the femoral head. The stiffness and pain were attributable to the soft tissue surrounding the femoral head taking the impact of motion, and also attempting to protect the fragile bone structure. Treating one aspect without the other would have been less successful.

The treatment techniques demonstrate the combined use of adult and pediatric techniques. The initial treatment included three adult techniques adapted to a child's body. These are excellent physical-therapy-type movements, because they invigorate the soft tissue as well as the energetic layers. The adult techniques emphasized manipulation of the soft tissue surrounding the femoral head, encouraging relaxation and an increase in the flow of qi and blood to the area. The points were chosen to tonify the underlying energetic framework at the organ, particularly kidney, level.

CHRONIC DIARRHEA

Child information: Three-year-old male, average weight and height.

Presenting symptoms: Abdominal distension, occasional pain prior to bowel movement, consistently loose stools, chronic pattern of diarrhea and foul gas.

History: Diarrhea pattern has been persistent since birth with occasional fluctuations; no significant response to various medical treatments.

Assessment: Shen: good; tongue: no coating, slightly red body; abdomen: tense, pain upon palpation at upper left quadrant; stool: foul odor, difficult, and takes a long time to pass.

TCM differentiation: Spleen-deficiency diarrhea.

FIRST CPM TREATMENT

Press rotate Spleen Meridian

Press rotate Kidney Meridian

Push (clear) Small Intestine Meridian

Press rotate Small Celestial Center

Rotate push Inner Eight Symbols

Push Three Passes

Push Below Ribs

Rotate push Abdomen

Press rotate Spinal Column

Push Bone of Seven Segments (upward)

Press rotate Tortoise Tail

Press rotate Bubbling Spring

Press rotate Ravine Divide

Press rotate Leg Three Miles

Push Celestial Gate

Push Water Palace

Press rotate Great Yang

HOME TREATMENT

Press rotate Spleen and Kidney Meridians

Rotate push Abdomen

TREATMENT RESPONSE

One week later the parent reported the child had no pain with bowel movement and had better frequency.

SECOND TREATMENT

The child had an upper respiratory infection; the tongue was pale with a white coating. The treatment was changed to include:

TO TONIFY KIDNEYS:

Press rotate Two Horses

Spinal pinch pull

Chafe, then rub hands together to warm Life Gate

Press rotate Meeting of Hundreds

TO DISPERSE WIND COLD:

Press rotate One Nestful Wind

Press rotate Welcome Fragrance

FOLLOW-UP

Treatments continued twice a week for four weeks, once per week for two weeks, and once every two weeks for seven weeks. After the fourth treatment there was a change in the loose stool, although it was still not consistent. After three more treatments the bowel movements were consistently regular. At this time the Chinese herbal formula Saussurea and Cardamon Combination was given in granular form to be taken 1 gram twice each day. After an additional four treatments there was an absence of symptoms. Six more treatments were given to reinforce the spleen function. A follow-up one year later confirmed no recurrence of diarrhea.

COMMENTS

This case well illustrates a spleen deficiency becoming chronic and very stubborn to resolve. It was surprising to note that the child did not present any major deficiency patterns other than tending to contract EPIs. When this occurred, EPI-related points were added to the treatment.

The major changes in the treatment plan included an emphasis, after the first treatment, on tonifying the kidney with Life Gate and Meeting of Hundreds; also, the short-term use of Chinese herbs after the sixth treatment produced a significant change in the pattern.

The parent played a significant role in the success of this treatment. She took an active interest in understanding the situation, learned massage techniques and used them daily at home, and brought the child for treatments consistently.

CANCEROUS TUMOR

Child information: Eighteen-month-old male, low-average weight and height.

Presenting symptoms: Side effects of radiation and chemotherapy.

History: Diagnosis of cancerous abdominal tumor at twelve months old. Initial exploratory surgery confirmed this and discovered that the tumor was inoperable due to location. Radiation began, and the treatment continued with ten courses of chemotherapy over a one-year period.

Assessment: The first pediatric massage treatment occurred between the fifth and sixth rounds of chemotherapy. The child was basically asymptomatic during these periods. The most obvious signs of imbalance were a slightly purplish vein at first-gate IFV; thrush around lips; and a noticeable lack of fullness and tone of muscles in general, the abdomen in particular.

TCM differentiation: Depletion of qi and blood; slightly deficient yin heat.

First CPM Treatment

Press rotate Spleen Meridian

Press rotate Kidney Meridian

Press rotate Two Horses

Rotate push Inner Eight Symbols

Push Three Passes

Rotate push Abdomen

Push Below Ribs

Press rotate along both sides of Spinal Column, especially Liver, Kidney, and Spleen Back Points

Press rotate Tortoise Tail

Press rotate Bubbling Spring

Press rotate Ravine Divide

Press rotate Leg Three Miles

Push Water Palace

Push Celestial Gate

Press rotate Great Yang

Press rotate Meeting of Hundreds

Home treatment

Press rotate Spleen and Kidney Meridians

Rotate push Abdomen

Treatment response

General improvement in disposition, appetite, and elimination.

Follow-up

Massage treatments continued approximately three times per month for a total of twenty-two treatments over a seven-month period. The protocol was adapted to the conditions as they changed. With presence of EPIs the basic protocol was modified to include press rotate Welcome Fragrance, Wind Pond, and Lung Back Point. With constipation (a chemotherapy side effect) push Wood Gate and push Bone of Seven Segments (downward) were added; with liver toxicity/stagnation (also a side effect of chemotherapy) push Liver Meridian was included.

Comments

In this case pediatric massage was used as a supporting therapy to primary intervention by Western medicine. The child was diagnosed and treatment began at twelve months. The first CPM treatment occurred at eighteen months, midway through the course of chemotherapy. The purpose of the massage was to mitigate the side effects of the drugs and surgery, provide ongoing support, and strengthen the child's immune system.

Between rounds of chemotherapy the child was fairly normal and asymptomatic, except for a tendency to contract EPIs. Depending on the type of drug used, he generally experienced seven to ten days of side effects after chemotherapy, including constipation/diarrhea, digestive/appetite disturbance, listlessness, and irritability. During these periods his tongue turned a deep, dark red with an occasional thick, dirty coating. His IFV showed a deeper purple and sometimes a greater length; his abdomen felt significantly weaker. These signs were not consistent after each chemotherapy treatment, however, possibly due to the different drugs used throughout the course.

The child's reaction to massage was generally good. During his postchemotherapy phases his parent reported noticeable improvements in recovery time.

The most effective techniques were on the abdomen. Rectifying the center is a general concept, but it allowed many aspects to be treated at once—and with this child, many things were going on. Attempting to treat the cancer or chase fleeting symptoms was less important than focusing on maintaining his center, so that his young body could process everything that was happening.

After the last round of chemotherapy the physician performed a final exploratory surgery and biopsy, which showed no cancer. The child's response to postsurgery massage was quick and obvious. The treatment protocol was adapted around the sensitive areas of the healing incision as well as sensitive areas in the back, which were in close proximity to the tumor.

This case is a good example of how Chinese and Western medicine can be used together. It would not be practical to treat a tumor with pediatric massage alone; however, it can be very useful to treat the whole child and not just the tumor.

The changes in the protocol reflected the changes in this child's condition. The regular nature of chemotherapy made these adaptations obvious. In other children the changes may be less dramatic, but the same process can be followed.

The mother was very involved in the ongoing care and treatment of the child. From the first treatment she learned some basic massage techniques, which she performed regularly. She was very committed to using massage and reported that she noticed her son's postchemotherapy recovery was quicker than the recoveries of other children receiving the same treatment in the hospital.

APPENDIX A

TECHNIQUE PRACTICE ON A RICE BAG

ONE OF THE DISTINGUISHING CHARACTERISTICS of tui na is the quality of the hand techniques used to manipulate qi in the body. As I discussed in chapter 6, Techniques, there are rigorous standards for evaluating the quality of these hand manipulations. The effectiveness of a pediatric massage is dependent on the skilled manipulation of the appropriate points. The development of skilled technique should be a high priority for any practitioner.

A characteristic that differentiates tui na hand manipulations from other massage techniques is the unique motion that the hand, wrist, forearm, and so forth produce in order to create a movement (or manipulation) at the point. The subtleties of these motions can range from simple to complex. The intricacies of each motion require practice and time if they are to evolve into smooth, relaxed, and effective manipulations. Indeed, this process cannot be overemphasized.

It is important to understand that learning technique from a book is limited at best. Books and videos can be good instructional aids; however, there is no substitute for proper guidance and supervision by a trained practitioner.

The traditional way to learn techniques is to practice the movements on a rice bag—a small cloth bag or pillow filled with rice—supervised by a teacher. Given the proper density of rice, such a bag closely simulates the feel of working on a human body. It also provides a good context to learn the techniques before using them on a patient. Dexterity and skill should be achieved on a rice bag and not at the expense of patients.

There is no exact size requirement for a rice bag. It should be large enough to allow

217

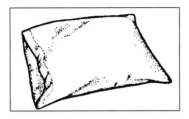

RICE BAG

full use of your hand to practice. An average-size bag measures eight inches by six inches, with approximately three inches of depth. The depth and density of the bag will be determined by how much rice you add—ideally, enough to form a dense, compact center that will allow a slight depression when you apply hand pressure. Too much rice will result in a bag that is too hard and has no give with pressure. Too little rice results in a bag that has no stable form, because the rice constantly shifts with pressure. The average-size bag contains approximately three pounds of rice.

Making a rice bag is fairly easy. Sew a small bag in the dimensions noted above, leaving a corner open. Fill the bag with rice and finish by closing the opening. Use a heavy-gauge thread and make the stitching strong. The bag should be sturdy, because it will need to endure repetitive motion and pressure. You can use almost any material; however, coarser and synthetic materials may be slightly irritating to your hand,

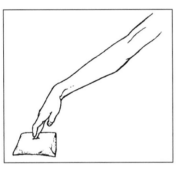

ARM ANGLE TO RICE BAG

due to the repetitive nature of the techniques. It is also possible to sew a "pillowcase" to fit over the rice bag, which lets you use a softer material and wash the outer case when necessary.

A simpler way to create a rice bag is to cut off the leg of a pair of pants, sew together one end, fill with rice, and sew the other end. Again, pay attention to the coarseness of the material.

Practicing on the rice bag is also fairly simple. Find a table of an appropriate height to work on. Ideally, you would use a massage table or something similar. Stand at the side of the table with the rice bag

directly in front of you. The ideal height of the table depends on your height. In the standing position, your arms should be relaxed and have a natural forty-five-degree-downward angle toward the bag (see diagram). If the table is too high your forearms will be parallel to the ground; if it is too low your arms will hang straight down, perpendicular to the ground. Both extremes are detrimental to good technique. You can raise the height of the rice bag by inserting thin books under it until its position is ideal. (Indeed, when you practice on the rice bag you can achieve an ideal rarely seen in an actual clinical situation.)

Using the descriptions of the techniques provided in chapter 6, approach the rice bag as if it were a human body, applying the technique to the "point." At first the movements may feel awkward and unnatural. This is why you train on a rice bag and not on a child. Work out the awkwardness and unnaturalness on the bag so that your technique is correct when you massage your patients.

Next, practice.

Then, practice.

Next, keep practicing.

There is no set training time that qualifies you as skilled, or ready to treat patients. It is a very individual process. Consistent, daily practice is recommended. To a skilled observer, it is obvious when someone "has it." Most people can also notice a difference in themselves. Refer to the four requirements of good tui na technique in chapter 6 (see page 40).

Practicing on the rice bag is also a good way to warm up before seeing your first patient of the day. This serves as preventive care for the practitioner, ensuring that your hands, wrists, and so on are properly prepared for the upcoming day. It is also a very good method for fine-tuning your techniques and connecting with the rhythm and vibration of the movement before touching a patient. Fifteen minutes of practice on a rice bag daily will reward you greatly.

Some students resist the process of practicing techniques on a rice bag. It takes time, patience, endurance, and attention to very subtle detail. Rather than approach practice as a boring but necessary evil, however, it is possible to use this experience as a meditation. This subtle shift in attitude may be crucial in your "getting it"—internalizing the intricate movements involved in tui na hand manipulations.

APPENDIX B

CHINESE PEDIATRIC MASSAGE CORE INFORMATION

A LARGE AMOUNT OF INFORMATION ON pediatric massage is contained in this book. Most practitioners will need access only to some basic techniques, points, and protocols to handle 80 to 90 percent of their pediatric cases. The remaining cases may require more advanced information.

As a guide to practitioners, the following techniques, points, and protocols can be considered the core information that you should learn.

Techniques
氣

Press

Press rotate

   Fingers 1, 2, 3

   Palm edge

   Lower palm

Fingernail press

Push

Chafe

Push apart

Rotate push

   Index and middle fingers

   Index, middle, and ring fingers

   Lower center palm

   Greater thenar eminence

Spinal pinch pull

Rub palms together

Points

Abdomen

Abdominal Center

Below Ribs

Bone of Celestial Pillar

Bone of Seven Segments

Bubbling Spring

Calm Breath

Celestial Chimney

Celestial Gate

Celestial Pivot

Chest Center

Curved Bone

Eight Sacral Holes

Elixir Field

External Palace of Labor

Five Digital Joints

Four Transverse Lines

Gallbladder Meridian

Great Hammer

Great Yang

Hall of Authority

Hundreds Worms Nest

Inner Eight Symbols

Inner Palace of Labor

Kidney Back Point

Kidney Line

Kidney Meridian

Kidney Summit

Large Intestine Meridian

Large Transverse Line

Leg Three Miles

Life Gate

Liver Meridian

Lung Back Point

Lung Meridian

Meeting of Hundreds

One Nestful Wind

Palmar Small Transverse Line

Ravine Divide

Six Hollow Bowels

Small Celestial Center

Small Intestine Meridian

Small Transverse Lines

Spinal Column

Spleen Back Point

Spleen Meridian

Stomach Back Point

Stomach Meridian

Three Passes

Three Yin Meeting

Tortoise Tail

Transport Earth to Water

Transport Water to Earth

Two Horses

Two Leaf Doors

Union Valley

Water of Galaxy

Water Palace

Welcome Fragrance
Wind Gate
Wind Pond
Wood Gate

Protocols

Abdominal pain

Asthma

Common cold

Constipation

Cough

Diarrhea

Earache

Enuresis

Fever

General health care

Headache

Milk or food stasis

Night crying

Poor digestion

Sore throat

Vomiting

APPENDIX C

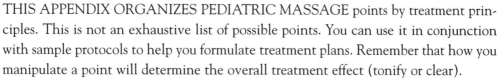

POINTS BY CATEGORIES

THIS APPENDIX ORGANIZES PEDIATRIC MASSAGE points by treatment principles. This is not an exhaustive list of possible points. You can use it in conjunction with sample protocols to help you formulate treatment plans. Remember that how you manipulate a point will determine the overall treatment effect (tonify or clear).

The categories in order are: Dispel Pathogenic Factors, Clear Heat, Tonify, Warm Yang and Dispel Cold, Promote Digestion and Remove Stagnation, Stop Diarrhea, Relieve Abdominal Pain, Promote Bowel Movement, Check Vomiting, Promote Urination, Regulate Lung Qi, Soothe Nerves, Resuscitate, Check Sweating, Harmonize Organs, Clear Meridians/Collaterals/Orifices, Activate Blood, Relieve Pain.

Dispel Pathogenic Factors
氣

Wind Cold

Bone of Celestial Pillar

Broken Sequence

Celestial Gate

Celestial Hearing

Central Hub

External Palace of Labor

Fontanel Meeting

Great Hammer

Great Yang

Hall of Authority

Lung Back Point

One Nestful Wind

Outer Pass

Three Passes

Two Leaf Doors

Wasp Entering Cave

Water Palace

Welcome Fragrance

Wind Gate

Wind Pond

Wind Heat

Bone of Celestial Pillar

Brain Hollow

Broken Sequence

Celestial Gate

External Palace of Labor

Fontanel Meeting

Great Hammer

Great Yang

Inner Palace of Labor

Kidney Line

Large Transverse Line

Lung Back Point

Lung Meridian

Metal Sound

Pool at the Bend

Six Hollow Bowels

Tip of Nose

Two Leaf Doors

Union Valley

Wasp Entering Cave

Water of Galaxy

Water Palace

Welcome Fragrance

Wind Gate

Wind Pond

Damp

Lesser Metal Sound

Spleen Back Point

Spleen Meridian

Three Passes

Three Yin Crossing

Phlegm

Celestial Chimney

Chest Center

Five Digital Joints

Four Transverse Lines

Inner Eight Symbols

Large Transverse Line

Lesser Marsh

Lesser Metal Sound

Lung Back Point

Lung Meridian

Metal Sound

Mountain Support

Outside Nipple

Palmar Small Transverse Line

Small Transverse Lines

Spleen Meridian

Two Horses

Two Leaf Doors

Water of Galaxy

White Tendon

Clear Heat
氣

Between Moments

Blue Tendon

Bone of Seven Segments

Bubbling Spring

Celestial Gate

Chief Tendon

External Place of Labor

Fish for Moon Under Water

Gallbladder Meridian

Great Hammer

Great Yang

Kidney Line

Kidney Meridian

Large Intestine Meridian

Lesser Marsh

Lesser Metal Sound

Liver Meridian

Lung Back Point

Metal Sound

Mountain Base

Nursing the Aged

Palmar Small Transverse Line

Passage Hub

Pupil Bone Hole

Six Hollow Bowels

Small Celestial Center

Small Intestine Meridian

Small Transverse Lines

Spinal Column

Spleen Meridian

Stomach Meridian

Ten Kings

Tip of Nose

Two Leaf Doors

Vast Pool

Water of Galaxy

Water Palace

Wind Pond

Wood Gate

Tonify
氣

Abdomen

Abdominal Center

Abdominal Yin Yang

Back Ravine

Bubbling Spring

Central Pivot

Elixir Field

External Place of Labor

Heart Meridian

Kidney Back Point

Kidney Meridian

Kidney Summit

Large Intestine Meridian

Leg Three Miles

Lumbar Back Point

Lung Back Point

Lung Meridian

Meeting of Hundreds

Monkey Plucks Apples

Nursing the Aged

One Nestful Wind

Ravine Divide

Small Intestine Meridian

Spinal Column

Spirit Gate

Spleen Back Point

Spleen Meridian

Three Passes

Tip of Nose

Transport Earth to Water

Transport Water to Earth

Two Horses

Wood Gate

Warm Yang and Dispel Cold
氣

Bone of Seven Segments

Celestial Gate to Tiger's Mouth

Elixir Field

External Palace of Labor

Kidney Meridian

One Nestful Wind

Spirit Gate

Three Passes

Tortoise Tail

Two Horses

Two Leaf Doors

Promote Digestion and Remove Stagnation
氣

Abdomen

Abdominal Center

Abdominal Yin Yang

Celestial Pivot

External Palace of Labor

Four Transverse Lines

Hand Celestial Gate

Inner Eight Symbols

Large Intestine Meridian

Large Transverse Line

Leg Three Miles

Six Hollow Bowels

Spirit Gate

Spleen Back Point

Spleen Meridian

Stomach Meridian

Transport Water to Earth

Two Horses

Vim Tranquillity

Wood Gate

Stop Diarrhea
氣

Abdomen

Abdominal Corner

Abdominal Yin Yang

Bone of Seven Segments

Bubbling Spring

Celestial Gate to Tiger's Mouth

Celestial Pivot

Elixir Field

External Palace of Labor

Front Mountain Support

Great Hammer

Kidney Back Point

Kidney Meridian

Large Intestine Meridian

Leg Three Miles

Liver Meridian

Meeting of Hundreds

Outer Pass

Ravine Divide

Small Celestial Center

Small Intestine Meridian

Spinal Column

Spirit Gate

Spleen Back Point

Spleen Meridian

Symmetric Upright

Three Passes

Tortoise Tail

Transport Earth to Water

Transport Water to Earth

Relieve Abdominal Pain
氣

Abdomen

Abdominal Corner

Abdominal Yin Yang

Below Ribs

Elixir Field

External Palace of Labor

Fish Border

Four Transverse Lines

Front Mountain Support

Inner Eight Symbols

Kidney Back Point

Large Intestine Meridian

Leg Three Miles

Liver Meridian

One Nestful Wind

Outer Eight Symbols

Spinal Column

Spirit Gate

Spleen Meridian

Stomach Meridian

Three Passes

Tortoise Tail

Transport Earth to Water

Two Horses

Water of Galaxy

Promote Bowel Movement
氣

Abdomen

Abdominal Corner

Arm Yang Pool

Bone of Seven Segments

Celestial Chimney

Front Mountain Support

Inner Eight Symbols

Large Intestine Meridian

Metal Sound

Outer Eight Symbols

Six Hollow Bowels

Spirit Gate

Spleen Meridian

Tortoise Tail

Transport Water to Earth

Union Valley

Check Vomiting
氣

Abdomen

Abdominal Yin Yang

Below Ribs

Bone of Celestial Pillar

Bubbling Spring

Celestial Chimney

Celestial Gate

Celestial Gate to Tiger's Mouth

Chest Center

Great Hammer

Inner Eight Symbols

Leg Three Miles

Lesser Metal Sound

Maternal Cheek

Pool at the Bend

Small Celestial Center

Spinal Column

Spleen Back Point

Stomach Meridian

Symmetric Upright

Transport Earth to Water

Union Valley

Promote Urination

Arm Yang Pool

Back Ravine

Elixir Field

Kidney Meridian

Sauce Receptacle

Small Celestial Center

Small Intestine Meridian

Winnower Gate

Regulate Lung Qi

Breast Root

Celestial Chimney

Chest Center

Four Transverse Lines

Inner Eight Symbols

Kidney Meridian

Leg Three Miles

Lesser Marsh

Lesser Metal Sound

Lung Back Point

Lung Meridian

Metal Sound

Outer Eight Symbols

Outside Nipple

Palmar Small Transverse Line

Small Transverse Lines

Two Horses

Two Leaf Doors

Vim Tranquillity

White Tendon

Wind Gate

Soothe Nerves
氣

Bamboo Gathering

Broken Sequence

Celestial Gate

Central Hub

Chief Tendon

Fish Border

Five Digital Joints

Ghost Eye

Great Yang

Hall of Authority

Human Center

Hundreds Worms Nest

Inner Palace of Labor

Kun Lun Mountains

Liver Meridian

Meeting of Hundreds

Mountain Base

Mountain Support

Nursing the Aged

One Nestful Wind

Pupil Bone Hole

Sauce Receptacle

Small Celestial Center

Subservient Visitor

Ten Kings

Tortoise Tail

Two Leaf Doors

Vast Pool

Water of Galaxy

Water Palace

Resuscitate
氣

Bamboo Gathering

Celestial Hearing

Five Digital Joints

Fontanel Meeting

Hall of Authority

Human Center

Imposing Agility

Old Dragon

Sweet Load

Ten Kings

Tiger Swallows a Prey

Two Leaf Doors

Vim Tranquillity

Water Palace

Check Sweating

Great Yang

Kidney Summit

Spleen Meridian

Harmonize Organs

Five Meridians

Inner Eight Symbols

Large Transverse Line

Spinal Column

Clear Meridians/Collaterals/Orifices

Auditory Palace

Bend Middle

Hundreds Worms Nest

Jawbone

Kun Lun Mountains

Lash Horse to Cross Galaxy

Subservient Visitor

Three Passes

Three Yin Meeting

Two Leaf Doors

Wind Gate

Year Longevity

Activate Blood
氣

Bridge Arch

Lesser Sea

Lumbar Back Point

Three Passes

Three Yin Meeting

Relieve Pain
氣

Abdominal Yin Yang

Before Vertex

Between Moments

Brain Hollow

External Palace of Labor

Four Whites

Jumping Round

One Nestful Wind

Outer Pass

Six Hollow Bowels

Union Valley

APPENDIX D

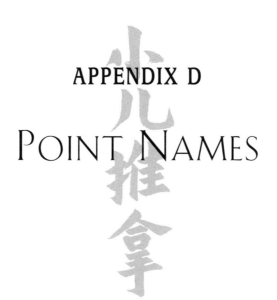

POINT NAMES

THIS APPENDIX CROSS-REFERENCES and sorts point names and information in three ways: by English name, by acupoint number, and by pin yin name.

ENGLISH SORT

English Translation	Pin Yin	Acu #	Region	Pg
Abdomen	Fu		Ant. torso	82
Abdominal Center	Zhong wan	CV 12	Ant. torso	82
Abdominal Corner	Du jiao		Ant. torso	82
Abdominal Yin Yang	Fu yin yang		Ant. torso	83
Arm Yang Pool	Bo yang qi		Arm	77
Auditory Convergence	Ting hui	GB 2	Head	102
Auditory Palace	Ting gong	SI 19	Head	102
Back Ravine	Hou xi	SI 3	Hand	56
Bamboo Gathering	Zan zhu	BL 2	Head	102
Before Vertex	Qian ding	GV 21	Head	103
Below Ribs	Xie lei		Ant. torso	83
Bend Middle	Wei zhong	BL 40	Leg	95
Between Moments	Xin jian		Head	103
Blue Tendon	Qing jin		Hand	56
Bone of Celestial Pillar	Tian zhu gu		Head	103
Bone of Seven Segments	Qi jie gu		Post. torso	88
Bountiful Bulge	Feng long	ST 40	Leg	95
Brain Hollow	Nao kong	GB 19	Head	104
Breast Root	Ru gen	ST 18	Ant. torso	83

English Translation	Pin Yin	Acu #	Region	Pg
Bridge Arch	Qiao gong		Head	104
Bright Eyes	Jing ming	BL 1	Head	104
Broken Sequence	Lie que	LU 7	Hand	56
Bubbling Spring	Yong quan	K 1	Leg	95
Calm Breath	Ding chuan	X 14	Post. torso	88
Celestial Chimney	Tian tu	CV 22	Ant. torso	84
Celestial Gate	Tian men		Head	105
Celestial Gate to Tiger's Mouth	Tian men ru hu kou		Hand	57
Celestial Hearing	Tian ting		Head	105
Celestial Pivot	Tian shu	ST 25	Ant. torso	84
Central Hub	Zhong chong	P 9	Hand	57
Central Islet	Zhong zhu	TW 3	Hand	57
Central Pivot	Zhong shu	GV 7	Post. torso	88
Central Treasury	Zhong fu	LU 1	Ant. torso	84
Chest Center	Dan zhong	CV 17	Ant. torso	85
Chief Tendon	Zhong jin		Hand	58
Curved Bone	Qu gu	CV 2	Ant. torso	85
Ear Wind Gate	Er feng men		Head	105
Earth Granary	Di cang	ST 4	Head	106
Eight Sacral Holes	Ba liao	BL 31–34	Post. torso	89
Elixir Field	Dan tian		Ant. torso	85
External Palace of Labor	Wai lao gong		Hand	58
Fire Palace (Inner Eight Symbols)	Li gong		Hand	58
Fish Back	Yu yao	X 5	Head	106
Fish Border	Yu ji	LU 10	Hand	59
Fish for Moon Under Water	Shui di lao yue		Hand	59
Five Digital Joints	Wu zhi jie		Hand	59
Five Meridians	Wu jing		Hand	60
Fontanel Gate	Xin men		Head	106
Fontanel Meeting	Xin hui	GV 22	Head	107
Four Transverse Lines	Sui wen	X 25	Hand	60
Four Whites	Si bai	ST 2	Head	107
Front Mountain Support	Qian cheng shan		Leg	96
Gallbladder Meridian	Dan jing	GB	Hand	60
Ghost Eye	Gui yan		Leg	96
Great Hammer	Da zhui	GV 14	Post. torso	89
Great Yang	Tai yang	X 1	Head	107
Hall of Authority	Yin tang	X 2	Head	108
Hand Celestial Gate	Shou tian men		Hand	61

English Translation	Pin Yin	Acu #	Region	Pg
Heart Back Point	Xin shu	BL 15	Post. torso	89
Heart Meridian	Xin jing	H	Hand	61
Human Center	Ren zhong	GV 26	Head	108
Hundreds Worms Nest	Bai chong wo	X 35	Leg	96
Imposing Agility	Wei ling		Hand	61
Inner Eight Symbols	Nei ba gua		Hand	62
Inner Palace of Labor	Nei lao gong	P 8	Hand	63
Inner Pass	Nei guan	P 6	Arm	77
Jawbone	Jia che	ST 6	Head	108
Jumping Round	Huan tiao	GB 30	Leg	97
Kidney Back Point	Shen shu	BL 23	Post. torso	90
Kidney Line	Shen wen		Hand	63
Kidney Meridian	Shen jing	K	Hand	63
Kidney Summit	Shen ding		Hand	64
Kun Lun Mountains	Kun lun	BL 60	Leg	97
Large Intestine Meridian	Da chang jing	LI	Hand	64
Large Transverse Line	Da heng wen		Hand	64
Leg Three Miles	Zu san li	ST 36	Leg	97
Lesser Marsh	Shao ze	SI 1	Hand	65
Lesser Sea	Shao hai	H 3	Arm	77
Lesser Metal Sound	Shao shang	LU 11	Hand	65
Life Gate	Ming men	GV 4	Post. torso	90
Liver Meridian	Gan jing	LV	Hand	65
Lumbar Back Point	Yao shu	GV 2	Post. torso	90
Lung Back Point	Fei shu	BL 13	Post. torso	91
Lung Meridian	Fei jing	LU	Hand	66
Maternal Cheek	Mu sai		Hand	66
Meeting of Hundreds	Bai hui	GV 20	Head	109
Metal Sound	Shang yang	LI 1	Hand	66
Mountain Base	Shan gen		Head	109
Mountain Support	Cheng shan	BL 57	Leg	98
Mute's Gate	Ya men	GV 15	Head	109
Nursing the Aged	Yang lao	SI 6	Hand	67
Old Dragon	Lao long		Hand	67
One Nestful Wind	Yi wo feng		Hand	67
Outer Eight Symbols	Wai ba gua		Hand	68
Outer Pass	Wai guan	TW 5	Arm	78
Outside Nipple	Ru pang		Ant. torso	86
Painful Point	Ah shi (Tian ying)		All regions	113

English Translation	Pin Yin	Acu #	Region	Pg
Palmar Small Transverse Line	Zheng xiao heng wen		Hand	68
Passage Hub	Guan chong	TW 1	Hand	68
Pool at the Bend	Qu qi	LI 11	Arm	78
Protruding Bone Behind Ear	Er hou		Head	110
Pupil Bone Hole	Tong zi liao	GB 1	Head	110
Ravine Divide	Jie xi	ST 41	Leg	98
Sauce Receptacle	Cheng jiang	CV 24	Head	110
Scapula	Jian jie gu		Post. torso	91
Sea of Blood	Xue hai	SP 10	Leg	98
Shoulder Bone	Jian yu	LI 15	Arm	78
Shoulder Well	Jian jing	GB 21	Post. torso	91
Six Hollow Bowels	Liu fu		Arm	79
Small Celestial Center	Xiao tian xin		Hand	69
Small Intestine Meridian	Xiao chang jing	SI	Hand	69
Small Transverse Lines	Sui heng wen		Hand	69
Snail Shell	Luo si		Hand	70
Spinal Column	Ji zhu		Post. torso	92
Spirit Gate	Shen que	CV 8	Ant. torso	86
Spleen Back Point	Pi shu	BL 20	Post. torso	92
Spleen Meridian	Pi jing	SP	Hand	70
Stomach Back Point	Wei shu	BL 21	Post. torso	92
Stomach Meridian	Wei jing	ST	Hand	70
Subservient Visitor	Pu can	BL 61	Leg	99
Suspended Bell	Xuan zhong	GB 39	Leg	99
Sweet Load	Gan zai		Hand	71
Symmetric Upright	Duan zheng		Hand	71
Tear Container	Cheng qi	ST 1	Head	111
Ten Kings	Shi wang	X 24	Hand	71
Three Digital Passes	Zhi san guan		Hand	71
Three Passes	San guan		Arm	79
Three Yin Meeting	San yin jiao	SP 6	Leg	99
Tiger's Mouth	Hu kou		Hand	72
Tip of Nose	Zhun tou	GV 25	Head	111
Tortoise Tail	Gui wei	GV 1	Post. torso	93
Transport Earth to Water	Yun tu ru shui		Hand	72
Transport Water to Earth	Yun shui ru tu		Hand	72
Two Horses	Er ma		Hand	73
Two Leaf Doors	Er shan men		Hand	73
Union Valley	He gu	LI 4	Hand	73

English Translation	Pin Yin	Acu #	Region	Pg
Upper Arm	Bi nao	LI 14	Arm	79
Vast Pool	Hong qi		Arm	80
Vim Tranquillity	Jing ning		Hand	74
Wasp Entering Cave	Huang feng ru dong		Head	111
Water (Inner Eight Symbols)	Kan gong		Hand	74
Water of Galaxy	Tian he shui		Arm	80
Water Palace	Kan gong		Head	112
Welcome Fragrance	Ying xiang	LI 20	Head	112
White Tendon	Bai jin		Hand	74
Wind Gate	Feng men	BL 12	Post. torso	93
Wind Mansion	Feng fu	GV 16	Head	112
Wind Pond	Feng qi	GB 20	Head	113
Winnower Gate	Ji men	SP 11	Leg	100
Wood Gate	Ban men		Hand	75
Yang Marsh	Yang xi	LI 5	Hand	75
Yang Mound Spring	Yang ling quan	GB 34	Leg	100
Year Longevity	Nian shou		Head	113
Yin Pool	Yin chi		Hand	75

ACUPOINT NUMBER SORT

Acu #	English Translation	Pin Yin	Region	Pg
BL 1	Bright Eyes	Jing ming	Head	104
BL 2	Bamboo Gathering	Zan zhu	Head	102
BL 12	Wind Gate	Feng men	Post. torso	93
BL 13	Lung Back Point	Fei shu	Post. torso	91
BL 15	Heart Back Point	Xin shu	Post. torso	89
Bl 20	Spleen Back Point	Pi shu	Post. torso	92
BL 21	Stomach Back Point	Wei shu	Post. torso	92
BL 23	Kidney Back Point	Shen shu	Post. torso	90
BL 31–34	Eight Sacral Holes	Ba liao	Post. torso	89
BL 40	Bend Middle	Wei zhong	Leg	95
BL 57	Mountain Support	Cheng shan	Leg	98
BL 60	Kun Lun Mountains	Kun lun	Leg	97
BL 61	Subservient Visitor	Pu can	Leg	99
CV 2	Curved Bone	Qu gu	Ant. torso	85
CV 8	Spirit Gate	Shen que	Ant. torso	86

ACU #	ENGLISH TRANSLATION	PIN YIN	REGION	PG
CV 12	Abdominal Center	Zhong wan	Ant. torso	82
CV 22	Celestial Chimney	Tian tu	Ant. torso	84
CV 17	Chest Center	Dan zhong	Ant. torso	85
CV 24	Sauce Receptacle	Cheng jiang	Head	110
GB	Gallbladder Meridian	Dan jing	Hand	60
GB 1	Pupil Bone Hole	Tong zi liao	Head	110
GB 2	Auditory Convergence	Ting hui	Head	102
GB 19	Brain Hollow	Nao kong	Head	104
GB 21	Shoulder Well	Jian jing	Post. torso	91
GB 30	Jumping Round	Huan tiao	Leg	97
GB 34	Yang Mound Spring	Yang ling quan	Leg	100
GB 39	Suspended Bell	Xuan zhong	Leg	99
GV 1	Tortoise Tail	Gui wei	Post. torso	93
GV 2	Lumbar Back Point	Yao shu	Post. torso	90
GV 4	Life Gate	Ming men	Post. torso	90
GV 7	Central Pivot	Zhong shu	Post. torso	88
GV 14	Great Hammer	Da zhui	Post. torso	89
GV 15	Mute's Gate	Ya men	Head	109
GV 16	Wind Mansion	Feng fu	Head	112
GV 20	Wind Pond	Feng qi	Head	113
GV 20	Meeting of Hundreds	Bai hui	Head	109
GV 21	Before Vertex	Qian ding	Head	103
GV 22	Fontanel Meeting	Xin hui	Head	107
GV 25	Tip of Nose	Zhun tou	Head	111
GV 26	Human Center	Ren zhong	Head	108
H	Heart Meridian	Xin jing	Hand	61
H 3	Lesser Sea	Shao hai	Arm	77
K	Kidney Meridian	Shen jing	Hand	63
K 1	Bubbling Spring	Yong quan	Leg	95
LI	Large Intestine Meridian	Da chang jing	Hand	64
LI 1	Metal Sound	Shang yang	Hand	66
LI 4	Union Valley	He gu	Hand	73
LI 5	Yang Marsh	Yang xi	Hand	75
LI 11	Pool at the Bend	Qu qi	Arm	78
LI 14	Upper Arm	Bi nao	Arm	79
LI 15	Shoulder Bone	Jian yu	Arm	78
LI 20	Welcome Fragrance	Ying xiang	Head	112
LU	Lung Meridian	Fei jing	Hand	66
LU 1	Central Treasury	Zhong fu	Ant. torso	84

Acu #	English Translation	Pin Yin	Region	Pg
LU 7	Broken Sequence	Lie que	Hand	56
LU 10	Fish Border	Yu ji	Hand	59
LU 11	Lesser Metal Sound	Shao shang	Hand	65
LV	Liver Meridian	Gan jing	Hand	65
P 6	Inner Pass	Nei guan	Arm	77
P 8	Inner Palace of Labor	Nei lao gong	Hand	63
P 9	Central Hub	Zhong chong	Hand	57
SI	Small Intestine Meridian	Xiao chang jing	Hand	69
SI 1	Lesser Marsh	Shao ze	Hand	65
SI 3	Back Ravine	Hou xi	Hand	56
SI 6	Nursing the Aged	Yang lao	Hand	67
SI 19	Auditory Palace	Ting gong	Head	102
SP	Spleen Meridian	Pi jing	Hand	70
SP 6	Three Yin Meeting	San yin jiao	Leg	99
SP 10	Sea of Blood	Xue hai	Leg	98
SP 11	Winnower Gate	Ji men	Leg	100
ST	Stomach Meridian	Wei jing	Hand	70
ST 1	Tear Container	Cheng qi	Head	111
ST 2	Four Whites	Si bai	Head	107
ST 4	Earth Granary	Di cang	Head	106
ST 6	Jawbone	Jia che	Head	108
ST 18	Breast Root	Ru gen	Ant. torso	83
ST 25	Celestial Pivot	Tian shu	Ant. torso	84
ST 36	Leg Three Miles	Zu san li	Leg	97
ST 40	Bountiful Bulge	Feng long	Leg	95
ST 41	Ravine Divide	Jie xi	Leg	98
TW 1	Passage Hub	Guan chong	Hand	68
TW 3	Central Islet	Zhong zhu	Hand	57
TW 5	Outer Pass	Wai guan	Arm	78
X 1	Great Yang	Tai yang	Head	107
X 2	Hall of Authority	Yin tang	Head	108
X 5	Fish Back	Yu yao	Head	106
X 14	Calm Breath	Ding chuan	Post. torso	88
X 24	Ten Kings	Shi Wang	Hand	71
X 25	Four Transverse Lines	Sui wen	Hand	60
X 35	Hundreds Worms Nest	Bai chong wo	Leg	96

PIN YIN SORT

Pin Yin	English Translation	Acu #	Region	Pg
Ah shi	Painful Point		All Regions	113
Ba liao	Eight Sacral Holes	BL 31–34	Post. torso	89
Bai chong wo	Hundreds Worms Nest	X 35	Leg	96
Bai hui	Meeting of Hundreds	GV 20	Head	109
Bai jin	White Tendon		Hand	74
Ban men	Wood Gate		Hand	75
Bi nao	Upper Arm	LI 14	Arm	79
Bo yang qi	Arm Yang Pool		Arm	77
Cheng jiang	Sauce Receptacle	CV 24	Head	110
Cheng qi	Tear Container	ST 1	Head	111
Cheng shan	Mountain Support	BL 57	Leg	98
Da chang jing	Large Intestine Meridian	LI	Hand	64
Da heng wen	Large Transverse Line		Hand	64
Da zhui	Great Hammer	GV 14	Post. torso	89
Dan jing	Gallbladder Meridian	GB	Hand	60
Dan tian	Elixir Field		Ant. torso	85
Dan zhong	Chest Center	CV 17	Ant. torso	85
Di cang	Earth Granary	ST 4	Head	106
Ding chuan	Calm Breath	X 14	Post. torso	88
Du jiao	Abdominal Corner		Ant. torso	82
Duan zheng	Symmetric Upright		Hand	71
Er feng men	Ear Wind Gate		Head	105
Er hou	Protruding Bone Behind Ear		Head	110
Er ma	Two Horses		Hand	73
Er shan men	Two Leaf Doors		Hand	73
Fei jing	Lung Meridian	LU	Hand	66
Fei shu	Lung Back Point	BL 13	Post. torso	91
Feng qi	Wind Pond	GB 20	Head	113
Feng fu	Wind Mansion	GV 16	Head	112
Feng long	Bountiful Bulge	ST 40	Leg	95
Feng men	Wind Gate	BL 12	Post. torso	93
Fu	Abdomen		Ant. torso	82
Fu yin yang	Abdominal Yin Yang		Ant. torso	83
Gan jing	Liver Meridian	LV	Hand	65
Gan zai	Sweet Load		Hand	71
Guan chong	Passage Hub	TW 1	Hand	68
Gui wei	Tortoise Tail	GV 1	Post. torso	93
Gui yan	Ghost Eye		Leg	96

Pin Yin	English Translation	Acu #	Region	Pg
He gu	Union Valley	LI 4	Hand	73
Hong qi	Vast Pool		Arm	80
Hou xi	Back Ravine	SI 3	Hand	56
Hu kou	Tiger's Mouth		Hand	72
Huan tiao	Jumping Round	GB 30	Leg	97
Huang feng ru dong	Wasp Entering Cave		Head	111
Ji men	Winnower Gate	SP 11	Leg	100
Ji zhu	Spinal Column		Post. torso	92
Jia che	Jawbone	ST 6	Head	108
Jian jie gu	Scapula		Post. torso	91
Jian jing	Shoulder Well	GB 21	Post. torso	91
Jian yu	Shoulder Bone	LI 15	Arm	78
Jie xi	Ravine Divide	ST 41	Leg	98
Jing ming	Bright Eyes	BL 1	Head	104
Jing ning	Vim Tranquillity		Hand	74
Kan gong	Water (Inner Eight Symbols)		Hand	74
Kan gong	Water Palace		Head	112
Kun lun	Kun Lun Mountains	BL 60	Leg	97
Lao long	Old Dragon		Hand	67
Li gong	Fire Palace (Inner Eight Symbols)		Hand	58
Lie que	Broken Sequence	LU 7	Hand	56
Liu fu	Six Hollow Bowels		Arm	79
Luo si	Snail Shell		Hand	70
Ming men	Life Gate	GV 4	Post. torso	90
Mu sai	Maternal Cheek		Hand	66
Nao kong	Brain Hollow	GB 19	Head	104
Nei ba gua	Inner Eight Symbols		Hand	62
Nei guan	Inner Pass	P 6	Arm	77
Nei lao gong	Inner Palace of Labor	P 8	Hand	63
Nian shou	Year Longevity		Head	113
Pi jing	Spleen Meridian	SP	Hand	70
Pi shu	Spleen Back Point	BL 20	Post. torso	92
Pu can	Subservient Visitor	BL 61	Leg	99
Qi jie gu	Bone of Seven Segments		Post. torso	88
Qian cheng shan	Front Mountain Support		Leg	96
Qian ding	Before Vertex	GV 21	Head	103
Qiao gong	Bridge Arch		Head	104
Qing jin	Blue Tendon		Hand	56
Qu qi	Pool at the Bend	LI 11	Arm	78

Pin Yin	English Translation	Acu #	Region	Pg
Qu gu	Curved Bone	CV 2	Ant. torso	85
Ren zhong	Human Center	GV 26	Head	108
Ru gen	Breast Root	ST 18	Ant. torso	83
Ru pang	Outside Nipple		Ant. torso	86
San guan	Three Passes		Arm	79
San yin jiao	Three Yin Meeting	SP 6	Leg	99
Shan gen	Mountain Base		Head	109
Shang yang	Metal Sound	LI 1	Hand	66
Shao hai	Lesser Sea	H 3	Arm	77
Shao shang	Lesser Metal Sound	LU 11	Hand	65
Shao ze	Lesser Marsh	SI 1	Hand	65
Shen ding	Kidney Summit		Hand	64
Shen jing	Kidney Meridian	K	Hand	63
Shen que	Spirit Gate	CV 8	Ant. torso	86
Shen shu	Kidney Back Point	BL 23	Post. torso	90
Shen wen	Kidney Line		Hand	63
Shi wang	Ten Kings	X 24	Hand	71
Shou tian men	Hand Celestial Gate		Hand	61
Shui di lao yue	Fish for Moon Under Water		Hand	59
Si bai	Four Whites	ST 2	Head	107
Sui heng wen	Small Transverse Lines		Hand	69
Sui wen	Four Transverse Lines	X 25	Hand	60
Tai yang	Great Yang	X 1	Head	107
Tian he shui	Water of Galaxy		Arm	80
Tian men	Celestial Gate		Head	105
Tian men ru hu kou	Celestial Gate to Tiger's Mouth		Hand	57
Tian shu	Celestial Pivot	ST 25	Ant. torso	84
Tian ting	Celestial Hearing		Head	105
Tian tu	Celestial Chimney	CV 22	Ant. torso	84
Tian ying	Painful Point (Ah shi)		All regions	113
Tian zhu gu	Bone of Celestial Pillar		Head	103
Ting gong	Auditory Palace	SI 19	Head	102
Ting hui	Auditory Convergence	GB 2	Head	102
Tong zi liao	Pupil Bone Hole	GB 1	Head	110
Wai ba gua	Outer Eight Symbols		Hand	68
Wai guan	Outer Pass	TW 5	Arm	78
Wai lao gong	External Palace of Labor		Hand	58
Wei jing	Stomach Meridian	ST	Hand	70
Wei ling	Imposing Agility		Hand	61

Pin Yin	English Translation	Acu #	Region	Pg
Wei shu	Stomach Back Point	BL 21	Post. torso	92
Wei zhong	Bend Middle	BL 40	Leg	95
Wu jing	Five Meridians		Hand	60
Wu zhi jie	Five Digital Joints		Hand	59
Xiao chang jing	Small Intestine Meridian	SI	Hand	69
Xiao tian xin	Small Celestial Center		Hand	69
Xie lei	Below Ribs		Ant. torso	83
Xin hui	Fontanel Meeting	GV 22	Head	107
Xin jian	Between Moments		Head	103
Xin jing	Heart Meridian	H	Hand	61
Xin men	Fontanel Gate		Head	106
Xin shu	Heart Back Point	BL 15	Post. torso	89
Xuan zhong	Suspended Bell	GB 39	Leg	99
Xue hai	Sea of Blood	SP 10	Leg	98
Ya men	Mute's Gate	GV 15	Head	109
Yang lao	Nursing the Aged	SI 6	Hand	67
Yang ling quan	Yang Mound Spring	GB 34	Leg	100
Yang xi	Yang Marsh	LI 5	Hand	75
Yao shu	Lumbar Back Point	GV 2	Post. torso	90
Yi wo feng	One Nestful Wind		Hand	67
Yin qi	Yin Pool		Hand	75
Yin tang	Hall of Authority	X 2	Head	108
Ying xiang	Welcome Fragrance	LI 20	Head	112
Yong quan	Bubbling Spring	K 1	Leg	95
Yu ji	Fish Border	LU 10	Hand	59
Yu yao	Fish Back	X 5	Head	106
Yun shui ru tu	Transport Water to Earth		Hand	72
Yun tu ru shui	Transport Earth to Water		Hand	72
Zan zhu	Bamboo Gathering	BL 2	Head	102
Zheng xiao heng wen	Palmar Small Transverse Line		Hand	68
Zhi san guan	Three Digital Passes		Hand	71
Zhong chong	Central Hub	P 9	Hand	57
Zhong fu	Central Treasury	LU 1	Ant. torso	84
Zhong jin	Chief Tendon		Hand	58
Zhong shu	Central Pivot	GV7	Post. torso	88
Zhong wan	Abdominal Center	CV12	Ant. torso	82
Zhong zhu	Central Islet	TW 3	Hand	57
Zhun tou	Tip of Nose	GV 25	Head	111
Zu san li	Leg Three Miles	ST 36	Leg	97

APPENDIX E

GLOSSARY OF CHINESE MEDICAL TERMINOLOGY

THE TECHNICAL TERMINOLOGY of traditional Chinese medicine varies from book to book, depending on the author and translation style. Following are definitions of TCM words and concepts as I have used them within this book.

Blood is yin in relation to qi (yang). A very dense and material form of qi provides nourishment, moistens tissues, and offers a material foundation for the body.

Clearing is a method of correcting an energetic excess through a treatment technique that lowers what is excessive, (for example, to clear the lung meridian of accumulated heat by using the push technique). Opposite of tonify. Synonyms: reduce, expel.

Cold—one of the eight principles—is an energetic quality manifesting in the body. Common attributes of cold include: cold sensations in the body, desire for warmth, contraction, and obstruction.

Congenital qi—one type of qi in the body—is the combination of qi inherited from both parents at conception. This is the foundation from which development and constitution derive. Synonyms: preheaven essence, prenatal qi, congenital essence.

Damp—one of the six pathogenic factors—is a yin pathogenic factor and refers to a damp quality of weather, living, or working environment. Damp is characterized by heaviness, stickiness, and slowed movement.

Defensive qi—one type of qi in the body—is responsible for the body's outer defense. It prevents external pathogenic factors from invading. Synonym: protective qi (pin yin: wei qi).

Deficiency—one of the eight principles—is yin relative to excess (yang). The term describes an energetic condition that is weak or has too little, less than enough (for example, deficiency in the lung meridian). Synonyms: vacuity, emptiness, insufficiency.

Dietary therapy—one of the therapeutic modalities of TCM—encompasses the use of daily foods to bring about an energetic result. Dietary therapy can play a very significant role in the overall treatment plan, because diet is such an integral aspect of daily living.

Essence is a very refined, primary foundation substance that supports the rest of the body's energetic functions. The term describes a combination of congenital and postnatal bases of life.

Excess—one of the eight principles—is yang in relation to deficiency (yin). This term describes an energetic condition that is overfull or too much (for instance, excess heat of the lung meridian). Synonyms: repletion, fullness.

Exterior—one of the eight principles—is yang in relation to interior (yin). The term refers to the outer and surface parts of the body: skin, body hair, muscles, superficial meridians.

External pathogenic invasion (EPI) describes the process of one or more pathogenic factors (wind, cold, dry, damp, fire, summer heat) penetrating the body's outer defenses. The quality of the combined pathogenic factors then influences the person's energetic pattern. Synonyms: pernicious influences, external evils.

Five phases is a theory that describes all phenomena as products of five basic phases of energetic development: wood, fire, earth, metal, water. In Oriental medicine five-phase theory is used to describe the energetic processes within the body. Synonym: five elements.

Fluid includes all of the normal liquid substances of the body: sweat, saliva, urine, and so forth. The main functions of fluids are to moisten, lubricate, and nourish.

Heat—one of the eight principles—is yang in relation to cold (yin). It is an energetic quality manifesting in the body. Heat indicators include: hot sensations in the body, elevated temperature, desire for coolness, burning pain.

Herbal therapy is the use of plant, animal, and mineral substances to influence the body's energetic nature. Application of herbal therapy can be internal or external.

Interior—one of the eight principles—is yin in relation to exterior (yang). The term describes the internal aspects of the body: organs, bone, internal channels.

Meridians are the pathways that transport qi, blood, and fluids throughout the body. Meridians function to connect all aspects of the body and maintain communication, forming an integrated whole. Synonyms: vessels, channels.

Original qi is a type of essence in the form of qi, rather than fluid. It is the foundation of both yin and yang qi in the body.

Pattern of disharmony is the term used to describe the energetic nature of an imbalance, illness, or disease. It refers to the relationship between energetic aspects in the body (for example, excessive liver yang qi).

Pin yin is one of several methods of translating Chinese characters into the alphabet system used in Western languages. Pin yin is currently the standard transliteration method used by the People's Republic of China.

Qi is a difficult word to translate into English (which is why *qi* is used instead of a translation). Qi is a very subtle vibration, or energy, that has not quite manifested into a material form; thus it has not been physically seen or measured. However, the effects and results of qi can be easily understood on a physical level. For example, applying finger pressure to an acupoint will generally result in both practitioner and patient experiencing some sensations of qi (tingling, warmth, movement, and the like). Synonyms: chi, ch'i, energy, ether, prana, breath, life force, vital force.

Qi gong is a method of exercise that strengthens the internal energetic aspects. Qi gong is internal relative to the external exercises of tai qi, martial arts, weight lifting, aerobics, and so on. Synonyms: chi kung, internal exercises.

Shen is the external manifestation of the internal essence. The term describes the overall physical, mental, and spiritual vitality of a person's energetic nature. Synonyms: spirit, mind, consciousness.

Stagnation is a sluggishness of movement. It may involve the movement of qi, blood, fluids, or materials through the body. Synonym: stasis.

Tai qi is the term for physical movements or exercises that enhance the flow of qi throughout the body.

Tonifying is a method of correcting an energetic deficiency through a treatment or technique that replenishes what is lacking (for example, to tonify deficient lung yin). Synonyms: supplement, reinforce, nourish, fortify.

Traditional Chinese medicine (TCM) is the reorganization of Chinese medicine by the

People's Republic of China government after the Communist Revolution in 1949. The development of TCM brought together many disparate segments of Oriental medicine into a unified system. TCM is the standard Oriental medical system used in the People's Republic of China, and is the predominant Oriental system in the United States.

Tui na—one of the three main branches of TCM—is the use of hand manipulations to influence energetic conditions in the body. Synonyms: massotherapy, Chinese medical massage.

Wade-Giles is a system for translating Chinese characters into the alphabet letters used in Western languages. Wade-Giles is currently not used in the People's Republic of China, but is still employed in Chinese communities outside the mainland (including Hong Kong and Taiwan). For example, *qi* is a pin yin translation, while *chi* is Wade-Giles.

Wind—one of the six external pathogens—refers to the energetic qualities of swiftness, movement, rapid onset, and changeability.

Yin/yang—a theory used throughout Oriental philosophy and medicine—describes all phenomena in the universe as pairs of complementary opposites. Although opposites, together yin and yang form a complementary whole and are interdependent. Nothing is either totally yin or totally yang.

Yang describes phenomena that are relatively more energetic. Yang corresponds to creation, activity, ascension, expansion, immateriality, heat, fire, summer, and so on.

Yin describes phenomena that are relatively more material. Yin corresponds to matter, structure, form, substance, contraction, descent, cold, water, winter, and so forth.

Ying qi is crucial to the formation of blood. The main function of ying qi is to flow throughout the meridians and blood vessels, nourishing the entire body. Synonyms: nutritive qi, construction qi.

APPENDIX F

CHINESE HERBS FOR PEDIATRICS

CHINESE HERBS CAN BE A VERY USEFUL adjunct to pediatric massage therapy. The combination of the two approaches may accomplish a quicker and more thorough recovery. In difficult cases the addition of herbal therapy can provide a daily method for home treatment. This appendix will present information on the use of Chinese herbs for pediatrics in three major areas: massage mediums, external applications, and internal formulas.

Proper therapeutic use of Chinese herbs requires specific training and knowledge. The purpose of this appendix is to present a broad outline of herbal uses for those already familiar with the guiding theories and principles of Chinese herbal medicine.

In general I will use the common names for herbs and formulas here. Common formula names are cross-referenced with pin yin names at the end of this appendix. See the appendix H, Bibliography, for Chinese herbal reference books.

Mediums
氣

Massage mediums serve dual functions in pediatric massage. First, they protect the child's delicate skin from the repetitive nature of the techniques. This is very important and should be incorporated in each massage. Second, you can choose a medium by considering its energetic properties. Mediums can be classified by their prevailing energetic nature and combined with a technique for therapeutic effect. For example, the warming nature of a medium is indicated for cold conditions; cooling mediums can be used in excess-heat conditions.

Sesame oil is the standard massage medium for most conditions, because it is slightly warming. Cool or cold water is the easiest medium for hot or excess conditions. Other massage mediums are listed with each protocol. These are optional and are not required for each condition, but may be useful in specific cases. For example, using a small amount of peppermint oil in some cool water may be very useful as a medium for the high fever, headache, and sore throat commonly seen with a summer EPI.

Juice Preparations

These mediums are produced by processing fresh, uncooked materials into a liquid form. Some juices can be extended by adding water.

Agastaches

> Preparation: Pound leaves and stalks, then squeeze.
>
> Properties: Pungent, slightly warm.
>
> Effects: Clear summer heat, resolve damp, rectify vital qi, harmonize middle burner.
>
> Conditions: Headache, dizziness, nausea, vomiting, chest oppression, itching from insect bites.

Chinese Hawthorne

> Preparation: Pound and crush.
>
> Properties: Sour, slightly warm.
>
> Effects: Resolve food stagnation.
>
> Conditions: Food stagnation, diarrhea, constipation.

Dandelion

> Preparation: Wash, clean, and crush.
>
> Properties: Sweet, bitter, and cold.
>
> Effects: Clear heat, detoxify, abate swelling, eliminate stagnation.
>
> Conditions: Scrofula, carbuncle, cellulitis, skin infections.

Egg White

> Preparation: Separate yolk from white.
>
> Properties: Sweet, salty, and placid.

Effects: Strengthen stomach/spleen, moisten skin and lung, abate swelling, relieve pain, smooth skin, clear pathogenic heat.

Conditions: Toothache; parotitis; mumps; scrofula; sore throat; cough; fever; skin infections, dryness, and poxes.

Garlic

Preparation: Peel, pound, and crush.

Properties: Pungent, warm.

Effects: Detoxify, warm middle burner, invigorate stomach.

Conditions: Common cold, cough, swellings, rashes.

Ginger

Preparation: Pound into pulp, filter juice, and add water.

Properties: Pungent, slightly warm.

Effects: Relieve exterior, disperse cold, warm middle burner, stop vomiting, smooth skin, warm yang.

Conditions: Common cold, stiff neck, headache, dyspnea, cough, abdominal pain, diarrhea, vomiting, abdominal distension.

Comments: Use in winter and spring.

Human Milk

Preparation: Obtain from a healthy woman.

Properties: Sweet, salty, and placid.

Effects: Tonify deficiency, benefit vital qi, clear heat, moisten dryness, tonify five organs, facilitate intestinal tract, nourish blood.

Conditions: Conjunctivitis; tic from wind; gastric-deficiency disturbance; malnutrition; abdominal pain; diarrhea; anuria; skin pain, itching, chapping, or dryness.

Comments: Fresh cow milk may be substituted.

Lotus

Preparation: Press.

Properties: Sweet, cold.

Effects: Clear heat, promote fluids, cool blood, resolve stasis.

Conditions: Skin diseases, poxes, and infections.

Comments: Use thick and tender roots; slippery and greasy.

Lotus Leaf

Preparation: Pound and crush.

Properties: Bitter, astringent, and placid.

Effects: Raise and circulate clear yang, clear summer heat, resolve stasis, stop bleeding.

Conditions: Rubella, pox, purpura.

Peppermint

Preparation: Pound leaves and stalks, then crush.

Properties: Pungent, cool.

Effects: Disperse wind, clear heat, relieve depressed qi, expel pathogenic factors from exterior, smooth skin.

Conditions: External wind heat, headache, stuffy nose, sore throat, toothache.

Comments: Use in summer.

Scallion

Preparation: Wash and press.

Properties: Pungent, warm.

Effects: Induce perspiration, promote yang, promote diuresis, smooth skin, dredge channels, activate circulation, dispel cold, relieve surface.

Conditions: Lower abdominal pain, abdominal pain, dysuria.

Comments: Dilute slightly; use in winter and spring.

Swine Bile

Properties: Bitter, cold.

Effects: Clear heat, relax bowels, abate swelling, eliminate stagnation.

Conditions: Dizziness, hypertension.

Comments: Fresh is preferable; reconstituted dried is usable.

Trichosanthes Fruit

Preparation: Peel skin, discard seeds, and crush.

Properties: Sweet, cold.

Effects: Moisten lung, large intestine, and skin; resolve phlegm; eliminate stagnation.

Conditions: Cough, chest pain and choking, breast swelling.

Water Chestnut

Preparation: Wash, break into pieces, and press.

Properties: Sweet, slightly cold.

Effects: Clear heat, improve eyesight, eliminate stasis, resolve phlegm.

Conditions: Spleen-deficiency fever, abdominal mass, jaundice.

Comments: Slippery and greasy.

Water Preparations

Soak herbs in warm or hot water; pungent warm herbs (such as ma huang or chrysanthemum) require twenty minutes; heat-clearing and detoxifying herbs (such as scute and coptis) need thirty minutes or more. Stir occasionally while soaking.

Chrysanthemum Flowers

Preparation: Steep.

Properties: Sweet, bitter, and placid.

Effects: Expel wind, clear heat, improve eyesight.

Conditions: Headache, fever, conjunctivitis, eye swelling and pain, dizziness, hypertension.

Cinnamon Twigs

Preparation: Steep.

Properties: Pungent, sweet, and warm.

Effects: Relieve muscles, induce perspiration, warm meridians, tonify yang.

Conditions: Common cold with fever, headache, chest oppression, dyspnea, back pain, diuresis.

Cold Water

Properties: Cool.

Effects: Clear heat.

Conditions: Fever.

Coriander Plant

Preparation: Steep.

Properties: Pungent, slightly warm.

Effects: Induce perspiration, promote eruptions, strengthen stomach, facilitate digestion.

Conditions: Measles, poxes.

Comments: Use especially when there is fever but no perspiration.

Lophatherum

Preparation: Steep.

Properties: Sweet, cold, and placid.

Effects: Clear heat from pericardium, eliminate vexation, promote diuresis, relieve thirst.

Conditions: Restlessness, fever.

Ma Huang

Preparation: Steep.

Properties: Pungent, slightly bitter and warm.

Effects: Induce perspiration, relieve exterior, quell asthma, promote diuresis.

Conditions: Headache, common cold, asthma, cough, rubella.

Musk

Preparation: Grind into powder, then steep.

Properties: Pungent, warm.

Effects: Open apertures, activate blood, dissipate stagnation.

Conditions: Coma, epilepsy, unconsciousness, abdominal mass, bruises.

Comments: Expensive.

Schizonepeta and Ledebouriellae

Preparation: Use 1:1; steep.

Properties: Pungent, warm.

Effects: Relieve exterior, expel wind, resolve damp, alleviate pain.

Conditions: Headache, common cold, throat swelling and pain, joint pain.

Tea

Preparation: Steep.

Properties: Bitter, sweet, and slightly cold.

Effects: Refresh mind, improve eyesight, clear heat, stop thirst, promote digestion, facilitate diuresis, abate fever.

Conditions: Fever.

Oil Preparations

You can create these mediums by soaking the material in oil, using powdered herbs in oils, or using ointments or other oil-based products (such as paraffin).

Carthamus

Preparation: Soak a small amount of carthamus in chicken fat and boil; use when cool.

Properties: Warm, acrid.

Effects: Moisturizing.

Conditions: Dry skin.

Chinese Ilex Oil

Properties: Bitter, astringent, and neutral.

Effects: Expel wind, tonify deficiency, moisten and nourish skin.

Conditions: Rubella, pain, itching and swelling of skin.

Glycerin

Properties: Sweet, neutral.

Effects: Tonify deficiency, moisten dryness.

Conditions: Stomach/spleen deficiency, dry skin.

Sesame Oil

Preparation: Room temperature.

Properties: Sweet, placid, and slightly warm.

Effects: Tonify deficiency, strengthen spleen, moisten dryness.

Conditions: Malnutrition, stomach/spleen deficiency, dry and rough skin.

Comments: The most common general-use pediatric massage medium.

External Formulas

The use of external applications of Chinese herbs in pediatrics has a long history; such preparations are commonly used by Chinese parents for folk treatment of simple conditions. Unfortunately, there is little written material on this subject. Still, the following are several applications and their actions.

Borneol and Borax

Preparation: Powder and mix with mild salt soup or chrysanthemum decoction.

Properties:

    Borneol: Acrid, bitter, and cool.

    Borax: Sweet, salty, and cool.

Effects: Open orifices; relieve heat, pain, and swelling; dry dampness; detoxify.

Conditions: Thrush, mouth ulcers.

Chinese Gall

Preparation: Powdered.

Properties: Sour, salty, and cold.

Effects: Astringe fluids.

Conditions: Night sweat.

Comments: Mix with vinegar into a paste; place on the navel before sleep.

Clove and Cinnamon Bark

Preparation: Powdered.

Properties: Acrid, warm.

Effects: Warm middle burner and kidney.

Conditions: Chronic diarrhea.

Comments: Apply to the navel.

Coriander

Preparation: Steam.

Properties: Pungent, slightly warm.

Effects: Promote eruption of measles.

Conditions: Measles.

Corydalis, Mustard Seed, Kansui, Asarum

Preparation: Powder, mix with ginger juice, form into a small cake, and add a clove to the center.

Properties:

Corydalis: Acrid, bitter, and warm.

Mustard seed: Acrid, warm.

Kansui: Bitter, sweet, cold, and poisonous.

Asarum: Acrid, warm.

Effects: Expel phlegm, resolve swelling, clear heat, move qi and blood, relieve pain, open chest.

Conditions: Asthma (especially during hot summer days).

Comments: Place on Lung Back Point, Gao huang shu (B 43), and Bai lao (X 16).

Fresh Scallion

Preparation: Mix with salt.

Properties: Pungent, warm.

Effects: Dispel cold.

Conditions: Dysuria.

Comments: Apply on the navel and lower abdomen.

Garlic

Preparation: Crush.

Properties: Acrid, warm.

Effects: Remove toxins.

Conditions: Chronic diarrhea.

Comments: Wrap in a packet and tie to around the navel or the sole of the foot.

Hibiscus

Preparation: Pound.

Properties: Pungent, neutral.

Effects: Cool blood, remove toxins, disperse swelling, control pain.

Conditions: Mumps.

Comments: Use fresh herbs; apply to parotid area.

Mirabilitum or Rhubarb

Preparation: Crush.

Properties: Bitter, cold.

Effects: Clear obstructions, drain heat.

Conditions: Food retention, abdominal distension.

Comments: Wrap herbs in a packet and tie around the navel. Monitor for skin irritation.

Purslane

Preparation: Pound.

Properties: Sour, cold.

Effects: Relieve swelling, clear heat.

Conditions: Mumps.

Comments: Use fresh herbs; apply to parotid area.

Ranunculus

Preparation: Pound with sugar.

Properties: Sweet, pungent, and warm.

Effects: Disperse heat and swelling.

Conditions: Pneumonia.

Comments: Use fresh herbs; apply to focus area of chest.

Scallion Stalk, Ginger, and Wheat Bran

Preparation: Heated.

Properties: Pungent, warm.

Effects: Dispel cold, warm middle burner.

Conditions: Food accumulation, internal cold.

Comments: Wrap in a packet while hot and apply to the navel; monitor for skin irritation.

Thrush Topical Powder

Preparation: Powdered (borax 3 grams, relagar 3 grams, camphor 1.5 grams, licorice 1.5 grams)

Properties:

Borax: Sweet, salty, and cool.

Relagar: Acrid, bitter, warm, and poisonous.

Camphor: Acrid, hot, and poisonous.

Licorice: Sweet, neutral.

Effects: Detoxify, clear heat, expel wind and damp, dry dampness.

Conditions: Thrush.

Comments: Apply topically.

Vegetable Sponge

Preparation: Pound.

Properties: Sweet, neutral.

Effects: Expel wind.

Conditions: Mumps.

Comments: Use fresh herbs; apply to parotid area.

Internal Formulas

This section is meant for practitioners who already have a firm background in using Chinese herbs. Many Chinese herbal references make only passing mention of pediatric usage. The exception to this is a recent excellent book by Bob Flaws, *A Handbook of TCM Pediatrics*. This book is for practitioners who have a complete crude or single-ingredient granule pharmacy and who can custom-prepare a formula. (See appendix G, Recommended Resources.)

The following appendix will be helpful as a quick index to standard formulas that may be available to practitioners in the form of prepared tablets, pills, or loose granules. While it may be ideal to be able to custom-prepare the individual ingredients in a formula, you can still achieve many benefits with some standard formulas available in prepared form.

The following formulas are grouped in categories roughly similar to the treatment protocols in this book. I have presented only the commonly used names of the formulas. A list of the common name, pin yin, and other names that each formula may be known by is located at the end of this appendix (see page 271). Experienced herbal practitioners should be well aware that some formulas with similar names in fact have different ingredients, depending on the manufacturer. Evaluate all formulas by their lists of ingredients, not their names. I have primarily used common formula names in this section, however the names of a few well-known products also appear here. These are Pill Curing, Andrographis Anti-Inflammatory Tablets, Forsythia Toxin Vanquishing Tablets, Succinum Dragon Embracing Pills, Laryngitis Pills, Autumn Pear Syrup, and Pulmonary Tonic Pills.

It is crucial to remember that children are not smaller versions of adults. This is particularly true in the administration of herbs. The dosage used for a particular child will depend on his or her age, growth and development, and degree of disharmony—as well as your own experience. A general standard for converting adult dosages for children is:

AGE	PERCENT OF ADULT DOSE
Newborns	$1/8 - 1/6$
6 months–1 year	$1/6 - 1/4$
1–3 years	$1/4 - 1/3$
3–7 years	$1/3 - 1/2$
7–10 years	$2/3$–full dose

Internal herbs can be taken in a variety of forms: teas, tablets, pills, capsules, powders, extracts, granules, and more. The availability of both ingredients and prepared products varies according to region and distributor. The formulas listed in this appendix may be available as prepared medicines (tablets, pills, or extracts), or you may need to create them from extracts or crude herbs.

Gaining children's compliance with taking Chinese herbs is not always an easy task. Different forms may be easier for children of different ages. Young infants may more easily take a liquid; small children may find powders or granules mixed in food easier; older children might be able to swallow small pills or capsules. It is useful if you know of several ways to administer similar formulas.

Practitioners without proper herbal training should not use these formulas without the guidance and supervision of a trained Chinese herbal practitioner.

ABDOMINAL DISTENSION

EXCESS/HEAT:

Agastache Combination

DEFICIENCY/COLD:

Saussurea and Cardamon Combination

ABDOMINAL PAIN

COLD:

Atractylodes and Hoelen Combination

Magnolia and Hoelen Combination

COLD/DEFICIENCY:

Aconite Restore Center Pills

Ginseng and Atractylodes Combination

FOOD RETENTION:

Citrus and Crataegus Combination

Pill Curing

SUMMER HEAT:

Agastache Combination

ASTHMA

HEAT:

Andrographis Anti-Inflammatory Tablets

Calm Asthma Pill

Protect Baby Powder

Return to Spring Powder

COLD:

Minor Blue Dragon Combination

KIDNEY DEFICIENCY:

Restore Kidney Function Pill

LUNG DEFICIENCY:

Jade Screen Combination with Cinnamon Combination

BLEEDING FROM NOSE (NONTRAUMATIC)

SPLEEN DEFICIENCY:

Ginseng and Longan Combination

Ginseng and Astragalus Combination

Ginseng and Atractylodes Combination

DEFICIENT HEAT:

Anemarrhena, Phellodendron, and Rehmannia Combination

DEFICIENT QI AND BLOOD:

Restorative Pills

BRONCHITIS, ACUTE

WIND/COLD:

Apricot Seed and Perilla Leaf Powder

Minor Blue Dragon Combination

WIND/HEAT:

Morus Leaf and Chrysanthemum Decoction

LUNG PHLEGM/HEAT:

Clear Lung Heat Pills

BRONCHITIS, CHRONIC

LUNG/SPLEEN DEFICIENCY:

Six Major Herbs Combination with Magnolia and Ginger Combination

LUNG/KIDNEY DEFICIENCY:

Perilla Seed Combination

CHICKEN POX

MILD:

Cinnamon and Astragalus Combination

Hoelen Five Herb Combination

Lonicera and Forsythia Combination

Protect Baby Powder

Return to Spring Powder

SEVERE:

Coptis and Scute Combination

COLIC

SPLEEN DEFICIENCY:

Peony and Licorice Combination

HEART FIRE:

Cinnamon and Dragon Bone Combination

Monkey Gallstone Powder

FRIGHT:

Protect Baby Powder

COMMON COLD

WIND/COLD:

Minor Blue Dragon Combination

WIND/HEAT:

Andrographis Anti-Inflammatory Tablets

Lonicera and Forsythia Combination

Morus Leaf and Chrysanthemum Decoction

CONSTIPATION

EXCESS HEAT:

Clear Lung Heat Pills

Forsythia Toxin Vanquishing Tablets

Guide Away Red Pill

DEFICIENT QI:

Four Major Herbs Combination

SPLEEN/LUNG DEFICIENCY:

Six Major Herbs Combination

CONVULSIONS, ACUTE

WIND/HEAT:

Lonicera and Forsythia Combination

WIND/COLD:

Pueraria Combination

SUMMER HEAT:

Elsholtzia Combination

PHLEGM:

Succinum Dragon Embracing Pills

PERICARDIUM AND YING HEAT:

Monkey Gallstone Powder

Zizyphus Combination

CONVULSIONS, CHRONIC

KIDNEY/SPLEEN YANG DEFICIENCY:

Stabilize the True Decoction

LIVER/KIDNEY YIN DEPLETION:

Precious Decoction for Ceasing Wind

COUGH

WIND/COLD:

Apricot Seed and Perilla Leaf Powder

Morus and Platycodon Combination

WIND/HEAT:

Laryngitis Pills

Morus Leaf and Chrysanthemum Decoction

LUNG HEAT:

Clear Lung Heat Pills

Clear Qi and Transform Phlegm Pills

Glehnia (Adenophora) and Ophiopogon Decoction

Succinum Dragon Embracing Pills

Bronchitis, Cough, Phlegm, Labored Breathing Pills

PHLEGM/DAMP:

Citrus and Pinella Combination

Ginseng and Perilla Leaf Combination

Monkey Gallstone Powder

Protect Baby Powder

YIN DEFICIENCY:

Autumn Pear Syrup

SPLEEN/LUNG DEFICIENCY:

Ophiopogon Combination

Pulmonary Tonic Pills

DELAYED FONTANEL CLOSURE

ESSENCE DEFICIENCY:

Golden Lock Consolidate Jing Pill

Diarrhea

Cold/damp:

Magnolia and Hoelen Combination

Heat:

Agastache Combination

Improper eating:

Citrus and Crataegus Combination

Fragile spleen:

Ginseng and Astragalus Combination

Ginseng and Atractylodes Combination

Six Major Herbs Combination

Stagnation:

Citrus and Crataegus Combination

Pill Curing

Digestion, Poor

Spleen damp:

Ginseng and Atractylodes Combination

Stomach/spleen deficiency:

Ginseng and Longan Combination

Six Major Herbs Combination

Earache

Cold:

Minor Bupleurum Combination

Liver fire:

Gentiana Combination

Yin deficiency:

Anemarrhena, Phellodendron, and Rehmannia Combination

Chronic:

Astragalus Combination

Edema

Wind:

Ma huang, Forsythia, and Phaseolus Decoction

DAMP HEAT:

Four Marvel Pill

KIDNEY/SPLEEN DEFICIENCY:

Restore Kidney Function Pill

Warm the Kidney Decoction

ENURESIS

WEAK CONSTITUTION:

Golden Lock Consolidate Jing Pill

Restore Kidney Function Pill with Reduce Urine Pill

SPLEEN/LUNG DEFICIENCY:

Ginseng and Astragalus Combination with Reduce Urine Pill

LIVER DAMP HEAT:

Anemarrhena, Phellodendron, and Rehmannia Combination

Gentiana Combination

EPILEPSY

PHLEGM:

Monkey Gallstone Powder

FEVER

WIND/COLD:

Cinnamon Combination

Pueraria Combination

WIND/HEAT:

Lonicera and Forsythia Combination

Morus Leaf and Chrysanthemum Decoction

LUNG HEAT:

Clear Lung Heat Pills

STOMACH/SPLEEN DEFICIENCY:

Ginseng and Astragalus Combination

SUMMER HEAT:

Agastache Combination

FLACCIDITY, FIVE KINDS OF

Ginseng and Astragalus Combination

Warm the Kidney Decoction

FURUNCLES

Forsythia Toxin Vanquishing Tablets

GENERAL HEALTH CARE

Four Major Herbs Combination

Six Major Herbs Combination

HEADACHE

WIND/COLD:

Cinnamon Combination

Pueraria Combination

WIND/HEAT:

Lonicera and Forsythia Combination

PHLEGM/TURBIDITY:

Citrus and Crataegus Combination

Monkey Gallstone Powder

HIVES

WIND/HEAT:

Tang Kuei and Arctium Combination

Wind/cold: Schizonepeta and Ledebouriella Combination

ILEUS

Agastache Combination

JAUNDICE

YANG JAUNDICE:

Capillaris Combination

YIN JAUNDICE:

Aconite Restore Center Pills

MALNUTRITION

FOOD STASIS:

Citrus and Crataegus Combination

SPLEEN DEFICIENCY:

Ginseng and Astragalus Combination

Ginseng and Longan Combination

QI/BLOOD DEFICIENCY:

Ginseng and Atractylodes Combination

Women's Precious Pills

MEASLES

PRIOR TO RASH:

Cimicifuga and Peucedanum Combination

Cimicifuga and Pueraria Combination

Lonicera and Forsythia Combination

AFTER RASH:

Aconite Restore Center Pills

Glehnia (Adenophora) and Ophiopogon Decoction

Warm the Kidney Decoction

REVERSE SYNDROME:

Guide Away Red Pills

MILK OR FOOD STASIS

DEFICIENCY/COLD:

Saussurea and Cardamon Combination

HEAT:

Agastache Combination

DAMP:

Citrus and Crataegus Combination

MUMPS

WIND/HEAT:

Lonicera and Forsythia Combination

Minor Bupleurum Combination

TOXIC HEAT:

Coptis and Scute Combination

NIGHT CRYING

DEFICIENCY/COLD:

Peony and Licorice Combination

Rehmannia Six Pill

HEART FIRE:

Cinnamon and Dragon Bone Combination

FRIGHT:

Protect Baby Powder

PARALYSIS

Astragalus and Peony Combination

PERSPIRATION

YANG DEFICIENCY:

Golden Lock Consolidate Jing Pill

EXCESS HEAT:

Guide Away Red Pill

DEFICIENCY FIRE:

Anemarrhena, Phellodendron, and Rehmannia Combination

PHLEGM CONDITIONS, CHRONIC

Citrus and Pinella Combination

Clear Qi and Transform Phlegm Pills

Succinum Dragon Embracing Pills

PNEUMONIA

Clear Lung Heat Pills

Succinum Dragon Embracing Pills

PROLAPSED RECTUM

STAGNANT HEAT:

Guide Away Red Pill

FRAGILE QI:

Ginseng and Astragalus Combination

RETARDATION, FIVE KINDS OF

KIDNEY/LIVER DEFICIENCY:

Restorative Pills

HEART/SPLEEN DEFICIENCY:

Ginseng and Longan Combination

RUBELLA

DURING ERUPTIONS:

Lonicera and Forsythia Combination

SKIN ERUPTIONS

Cimicifuga and Peucedanum Combination

Cimicifuga and Pueraria Combination

Forsythia Toxin Vanquishing Tablets

SORE THROAT

Morus Leaf and Chrysanthemum Decoction

STIFFNESS, FIVE KINDS OF

Ginseng and Aconite Decoction

Tang Kuei and Jujube Combination

SWOLLEN GUMS

Guide Away Red Pills

TEETHING OR TOOTHACHE

DEFICIENCY:

Peony and Licorice Combination

Zizyphus Combination

THRUSH

EXCESS FIRE:

Return to Spring Powder

Six Miracle Pills

DEFICIENCY FIRE:

Anemarrhena, Phellodendron, and Rehmannia Combination

Rehmannia Six Pill

URINATION, FREQUENT

KIDNEY DEFICIENCY:

Warm the Kidney Decoction

URINE RETENTION

QI DEFICIENCY:

Ginseng and Atractylodes Combination

DAMP/HEAT:

Gentiana Combination

VOMITING

WIND/COLD:

Pueraria Combination

WIND/HEAT:

Agastache Combination

ABNORMAL DIET:

Citrus and Crataegus Combination

STOMACH HEAT:

Agastache Combination

STOMACH COLD:

Aconite Restore Center Pills

Dioscorea Combination

Six Major Herbs Combination

FLAMING DEFICIENT YIN FIRE:

Glehnia (Adenophora) and Ophiopogon Decoction

WHOOPING COUGH

WIND/COLD:

Minor Blue Dragon Combination

WIND/HEAT:

Morus Leaf and Chrysanthemum Decoction

Morus and Platycodon Combination

Protect Baby Powder

Return to Spring Powder

LUNG PHLEGM/FIRE RETENTION:

Monkey Gallstone Powder

DEFICIENT LUNG:

Pulmonary Tonic Pills

DEFICIENT STOMACH/SPLEEN:

Minor Bupleurum with Pinella and Magnolia Combination

LUNG YIN INJURY:

Ophiopogon Combination

Chinese Herb Reference List
氣

The formulas mentioned above are included here for reference purposes. Each entry is listed under its commonly used name, followed by the pin yin (in parentheses), as well as the English translation and any other known name. The bibliography lists these common herbal reference books for more information: Bensky (1986, 1990); Cao (1990); Chen (1992); Dharmananda (1992); Flaws (1997); Fratkin (1986); Hsu (1997); Naeser (1993); Wiseman (1985); Yeung (1985); Zhu (1989).

Aconite Restore Center Pills; (Fu zi li zhong wan); Prepared Aconite Pill to Regulate the Middle.

Aconite, Ginger, and Licorice Combination; (Si ni tang); Frigid Extremities Decoction.

Agastache Combination; (Huo xiang zheng qi san); Agastache Powder to Rectify the Qi.

Andrographis Anti-Inflammatory Tablets; (Chuan xin lian kang yan pian).

Anemarrhena, Phellodendron, and Rehmannia Combination; (Zi bo ba wei wan, or Zhi bai di huang wan).

Apricot Seed and Perilla Leaf Powder; (Xing su san).

Astragalus and Atractylodes Combination; (Qing shu yi qi tang); Clear Summer Heat and Tonify Qi Decoction.

Astragalus and Peony Combination; (Bu yang huan wu tang); Paralysis Decoction; Tonify Yang to Restore Five Tenths Decoction.

Astragalus Combination; (Huang qi jian zhong tang); Astragalus Decoction to Construct the Middle.

Atractylodes and Hoelen Combination; (Ling gui zhu gan tang); Poria, Cinnamon Twig, Atractylodes, and Licorice Combination.

Autumn Pear Syrup; (Qiu li gao).

Bronchitis, Cough, Phlegm, Labored Breathing Pills; (Qi guan yan ke sou tan chuan wan); Chi Kuan Yen Pills.

Bupleurum and Cinnamon Combination; (Chai hu gui zhi tang).

Calm Asthma Pill; (Ding chuan wan); Arrest Wheezing Decoction; Ma huang and Ginkgo Combination.

Capillaris Combination; (Yin chen hao tang).

Cattle Gallstone Pill to Clear Heart; (Niu huang qing xin wan); Bos and Musk Combination.

Cimicifuga and Peucedanum Combination; (Xuan du fa biao tang); Dissipate Toxin and Release Exterior Decoction.

Cimicifuga and Pueraria Combination; (Sheng ma ge gen tang).

Cinnamon and Astragalus Combination; (Gui zhi jia huang qi tang).

Cinnamon and Dragon Bone Combination; (Gui zhi jia long gu mu li tang).

Cinnamon Combination; (Gui zhi tang).

Citrus and Crataegus Combination; (Bao he wan); Protect Harmony Pill.

Citrus and Pinella Combination; (Er chen tang); Two-Cured Decoction.

Clear Lung Heat Pills; (Qing fei yi huo pian).

Clear Qi and Transform Phlegm Pills; (Qing qi hua tan wan).

Conduct Perverse Qi Downward, Resolve Damp Phlegm Decoction; (San zi yang qin tang); Three Seed Decoction to Nourish One's Parents.

Coptis and Rhubarb Combination; (San huang xie xin tang).

Coptis and Scute Combination; (Huang lian jie du tang); Coptis Relieve Toxins Decoction.

Dioscorea Combination; (Szu shen tang).

Elsholtzia Combination; (Xiang ru san).

Forsythia Toxin Vanquishing Tablets; (Lian qiao bai du pian).

Four Major Herbs Combination; (Si jun zi tang); Four Gentleman Decoction.

Four Marvel Pill; (Si miao wan).

Gentiana Combination; (Long dan xie gan wan); Gentiana Liver Draining Pills.

Ginseng and Aconite Decoction; (Shen fu tang).

Ginseng and Astragalus Combination; (Bu zhong yi qi wan); Tonify Middle and Augment Qi Decoction.

Ginseng and Atractylodes Combination; (Shen ling bai zhu san); Codonopsis (or Ginseng), Hoelen, and Atractylodes Pills.

Ginseng and Ginger Combination; (Ren shen tang).

Ginseng and Gypsum Combination; (Bai hu jia ren shen tang); White Tiger plus Ginseng Decoction.

Ginseng and Longan Combination; (Gui pi wan); Restore Spleen Decoction; Nourish Spleen Pills.

Ginseng and Perilla Leaf Combination; (Shen su yin).

Glehnia (Adenophora) and Ophiopogon Decoction; (Sha shen mai men dong tang).

Golden Lock Consolidate Jing Pill; (Jin suo gu jing wan); Metal Lock Pill to Stabilize Essence; Lotus Stamen Combination.

Guide Away Red Pills; (Dao chi pian); Rehmannia and Akebia Combination.

Hoelen Five Herb Combination; (Wu ling san); Five Ingredient Powder with Poria.

Jade Screen Combination; (Yu ping feng san); Siler and Astragalus Combination.

Laryngitis Pills; (Hou yan wan).

Lepidium and Jujube Combination; (Ting li da zao xie fei tang); Descurainia and Jujube Decoction to Drain Lungs.

Lonicera and Forsythia Combination; (Yin qiao san); Yin Chiao Tablets; Honeysuckle and Forsythia Powder.

Ma huang, Forsythia, and Phaseolus Decoction; (Ma huang lian qiao qi xiao dou tang).

Magnolia and Ginger Combination; (Ping wei san); Calm the Stomach Powder.

Magnolia and Hoelen Combination; (Wei ling tang); Calm Stomach and Poria Combination.

Minor Blue Dragon Combination; (Xiao qing long tang).

Minor Bupleurum Combination; (Xiao chai hu tang).

Minor Cinnamon and Peony Combination; (Xiao jian zhong tan); Minor Construct the Middle Decoction.

Monkey Gallstone Powder; (Hou zao san); Hou Tsao Powder.

Morus and Platycodon Combination; (Dun sou san).

Morus Leaf and Chrysanthemum Decoction; (Sang ju yin or Sang ju gan mao pian).

Ophiopogon Combination; (Mai men dong tang).

Peony and Licorice Combination; (Shao yao gan cao tang).

Perilla Seed Combination; (Su zi jiang qi tang); Perilla Fruit Decoction for Directing Qi Downward.

Pill Curing; (Kang ning wan); Healthy and Peaceful Pill.

Pinella and Magnolia Combination; (Ban xia hou pu tang).

Precious Decoction for Ceasing Wind; (Da ding feng zhu); Major Arrest Wind Pearl.

Protect Baby Powder; (Bao ying dan); Po ying; Bo ying.

Pueraria Combination; (Ge gen tang); Kudzu Combination.

Pulmonary Tonic Pills; (Li fei tang yi pian); Benefit Lungs Tablets.

Reduce Urine Pill; (Suo quan wan); Shut Sluice Pill.

Rehmannia Eight Combination; (Ba wei di huang wan).

Rehmannia Six Pill; (Liu wei di huang wan).

Restorative Pills; (He che da zao wan).

Restore Kidney Function Pill; (Jin gui shen qi wan).

Return to Spring Powder; (Hui chun dan); Hui Chun Powder.

Saussurea and Areca Seed Combination; (Mu xiang bing lang wan); Aucklandia and Betel Nut Pill.

Saussurea and Cardamon Combination; (Xiang sha liu jun zi wan); Six Gentlemen with Aucklandia and Amomum Pill.

Schizonepeta and Ledebouriella Combination; (Jing feng bai du san); Schizonepeta and Ledebouriella Powder to Overcome Pathogenic Influences.

Six Major Herbs Combination; (Liu jun zi tang); Six Gentlemen Tea.

Six Miracle Pills; (Liu shen wan); Liu Shen Pills.

Stabilize the True Decoction; (Gu zhen tang).

Succinum Dragon Embracing Pills; (Hu po bao long wan).

Supplemented Saussurea and Coptis Tablets; (Qing fei yi huo pian).

Tang Kuei and Arctium Combination; (Xiao feng san); Eliminate Wind Powder.

Tang Kuei and Jujube Combination; (Dang gui si ni tang); Tang kuei Decoction for Frigid Extremities.

Warm the Kidney Decoction; (Zhen wu tang); Vitality Combination; True Warrior Decoction.

Women's Precious Pills; (Fu ke ba zhen wan); Gynecology Eight Jewel Pills.

Zizyphus Combination; (Suan zao ren tang); Sour Jujube Decoction.

APPENDIX G

RECOMMENDED RESOURCES

THE FOLLOWING RESOURCES ARE available for those interested in expanding their understanding of Chinese pediatric massage and the Chinese medicine approach to pediatrics in general.

Chinese Pediatric Massage
氣

Videos

Cline, Kyle. *Chinese Peidatric Massage—Practitioner's Reference Video*. Portland, Oreg.: Institute for Traditional Medicine, 1993.

————. *Introduction to Chinese Pediatric Massage*. Portland, Oreg.: Institute for Traditional Medicine, 1993. (A thirty minute introduction that includes demonstrations and interviews with parents who use the massage.)

————. *A Parent's Guide to Chinese Pediatric Massage Reference Video*. Portland, Oreg.: Institute for Traditional Medicine, 1994.

————. *Colic Relief: A Chinese Pediatric Massage Approach*. Portland, Oreg.: Institute for Traditional Medicine, 1996.

Books

Cline, Kyle. *Colic Relief: A Chinese Pediatric Massage Approach.* Portland, Oreg.: Institute for Traditional Medicine, 1996.

————. *Chinese Massage for Infants and Children.* Rochester, Vt.: Healing Arts Press, 1999. (Intended for parents interested in using pediatric massage.)

Chinese Medicine and Pediatrics
氣

Flaws, Bob. *Food, Phlegm & Pediatric Diseases* (pamphlet). Boulder, Colo.: Blue Poppy Press. (Information on diet and children.)

————. *Keeping Your Child Healthy with Chinese Medicine: A Parent's Guide to the Care & Prevention of Common Childhood Diseases.* Boulder, Colo.: Blue Poppy Press, 1996.

————. *A Handbook of TCM Pediatrics.* Boulder, Colo.: Blue Poppy Press, 1997.

Wolfe, Honora. *How to Have a Healthy Pregnancy, Healthy Birth.* Boulder, Colo.: Blue Poppy Press, 1993.

The Institute for Traditional Medicine can be reached at 1-800-544-7504. The Blue Poppy Press can be reached at 1-800-487-9296.

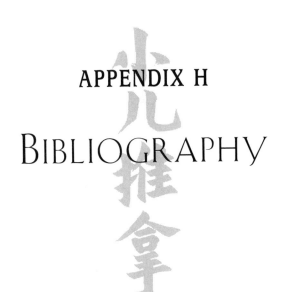

APPENDIX H

BIBLIOGRAPHY

Primary Sources
氣

English Language

Cao Ji-ming et al., eds. *Essentials of Traditional Chinese Pediatrics*. Beijing: Foreign Languages Press, 1990.

Fan Ya-li. *Chinese Pediatric Massage Therapy*. Boulder, Colo.: Blue Poppy Press, 1994.

Flaws, Bob. Turtle Tails and Other Tender Mercies: Traditional Chinese Pediatrics. Boulder, Colo.: Blue Poppy Press, 1985.

———. *A Handbook of TCM Pediatrics*. Boulder, Colo.: Blue Poppy Press, 1997.

Luan Chang-ye. *Infantile Tuina Therapy*. Beijing: Foreign Languages Press, 1989.

Sun Cheng-nan, ed. *Chinese Massage Therapy*. Jinan, China: Shandong Science and Technology Press, 1990.

Tiquia, Rey. *Chinese Infant Massage*. Richmond, Victoria, Aust.: Greenhouse Publications, Ltd., 1986.

Xiao Shu-qin. *Pediatric Bronchitis: Its TCM Cause, Diagnosis, Treatment and Prevention*. Boulder, Colo.: Blue Poppy Press, 1991.

Zhang En-qin, ed. *Chinese Massage*. Shanghai: Publishing House of Shanghai College of Traditional Chinese Medicine, 1990.

Chinese Language

俞大方 1989 推拿学 上海科学技术出版社　　　上海中国

金义成 1988 小儿推拿 上海科学技术文献出版社　上海中国

张思勤 1990 中国推拿 上海中医学院出版社出版 上海中国

孙承南 1989 齐鲁推拿医术　山东新华印刷厂印刷　山东中国

单吉平　张守杰 1987　　　单氏小儿推拿

　　　　上海第二医科大学附属瑞金医院中医科　上海中国

Secondary Sources
氣

Bensky, Dan. *Chinese Herbal Medicine Materia Medica.* Seattle: Eastland Press, 1986.

Bensky, Dan, and Randall Barolet. *Chinese Herbal Medicine: Formulas and Strategies.* Seattle: Eastland Press, 1990.

Cao Guo-liang. *Essentials of Tuinaology: Chinese Medical Massage and Manipulation.* Hilo, Hawaii: Cao's Fire Dragon, 1988.

Chen Ze-lin, and Chen Mei-fang. *A Comprehensive Guide to Chinese Herbal Medicine.* Long Beach, Calif.: Oriental Healing Arts Institute, 1992.

Cheng Xin-nong, ed. *Chinese Acupuncture and Moxibustion.* Beijing: People's Medical Publishing House, 1987.

Cui Yue-li. *The Chinese-English Medical Dictionary.* Beijing: People's Medical Publishing House, 1987.

Dharmananda, Subhuti. *Chinese Herbology.* Portland, Oreg.: Institute for Traditional Medicine, 1992.

Ellis, Andrew. *Grasping the Wind.* Brookline, Mass.: Paradigm Publications, 1989.

Fratkin, Jake. *Chinese Herbal Patent Formulas.* Santa Fe: SHYA Publications, 1986.

Hsu, Hong-yen. *Oriental Materia Medica: A Concise Guide.* Long Beach, Calif.: Oriental Healing Arts Institute, 1986.

————. *Commonly Used Chinese Herb Formulas.* Long Beach, Calif.: OHAI Press, 1997.

Lade, A. R. *Chinese Massage: A Handbook of Therapeutic Massage.* Vancouver: Hartley and Marks, 1987.

Maciocia, Giovanni. *The Foundations of Chinese Medicine.* New York: Churchill Livingston, 1989.

Naeser, Margaret. *Outline Guide to Chinese Herbal Patent Medicines in Pill Form.* Boston: Boston Chinese Medicine, 1993.

Sun Shu-chun. *Atlas of Therapeutic Motion for Treatment and Health.* Beijing: Foreign Languages Press, 1989.

Taber, Clarence. *Taber's Cyclopedic Medical Dictionary.* Philadelphia: F. A. Davis, 1989.

Unschuld, Paul. *Medicine in China: A History of Ideas.* Berkeley: University of California Press, 1985.

Wiseman, Nigel. *Fundamentals of Chinese Medicine.* Brookline, Mass.: Paradigm Publications, 1985.

Wu Jing-ying. *A Chinese-English Dictionary.* Beijing: Commercial Business Printing, 1989.

Xie Zhu-fan. *Dictionary of Traditional Chinese Medicine.* Hong Kong: The Commercial Press, Ltd., 1984.

Yeung Him-che. *Handbook of Chinese Herbs and Formulas.* Los Angeles: Institute of Chinese Medicine, 1985.

Zhu Chun-han. *Clinical Handbook of Prepared Chinese Medicines.* Brookline, Mass.: Paradigm Publications, 1989.

INDEX A

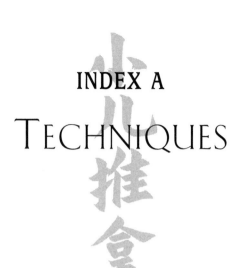

Techniques

INDEX B

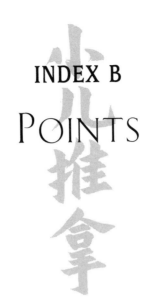

POINTS

INDEX C
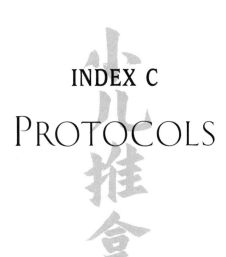
PROTOCOLS

INDEX D

INTERNAL HERBAL FORMULAS

NOTES

NOTES